THE
STRENGTH &
CONDITIONING
BIBLE

HOW TO TRAIN LIKE AN ATHLETE

NICK GRANTHAM

BLOOMSBURY

LONDON · NEW DELHI · NEW YORK · SYDNEY

Bloomsbury Sport
An imprint of Bloomsbury Publishing Plc

50 Bedford Square   1385 Broadway
London   New York
WC1B 3DP   NY 10018
UK   USA

www.bloomsbury.com

First published 2015

British Library Cataloguing-in-Publication Data
A catalogue record for this book is available from the British Library.

Library of Congress Cataloguing-in-Publication data has been applied for.

ISBN: PB: 978-1-4729-0897-1
         ePDF: 978-1-4729-0899-5
         ePub: 978-1-4729-0898-8

10 9 8 7 6 5 4 3 2 1

Typeset in Raleway by seagulls.net
Printed and bound in China by Toppan Leefung Printing

CONTENTS

To my wife Kate and our children Erin and Joe.

To my mum, dad and brothers.

To all of my mentors, colleagues and friends in the profession and to all the athletes and coaches, both past and present, that I've worked with over the last 18 years, thank you. You have all helped me form my views and beliefs and become the coach I am today.

ACKNOWLEDGEMENTS

This is a great opportunity for me to thank a number of people who have been instrumental in the completion of this book. First, I have to thank everyone at Bloomsbury for giving me this opportunity and taking a chance on a first-time writer.

To Kirsty Schaper, Sarah Cole and Jenni Davis, who helped me take this book from its initial conception to the final print.

Also to Newcastle University for providing the venue for the photo shoot and the models Jane Jones, Beth Johnsen, Jordan Wallace and Richard Eaton.

Along with those directly involved in the completion of this book, I would also like to thank the coaches, athletes, scientists and educators who I've worked with during the last 18 years and who have influenced me throughout my career. This book is really written by you.

Nick Grantham

FOREWORD

■ **This is not a book written by an Internet expert.** This is a book written by a real coach who trains real people.

I first worked with Nick in 2003 at the English Institute of Sport and I've continued to track his progress for more than a decade. I know that this book condenses, refines and delivers the knowledge and experience of one of the UK's leading hands-on strength and conditioning coaches.

Nick's track record speaks for itself. He's spent almost 20 years working behind the scenes in high-performance sport, coaching athletes from 35 different sports, including five Paralympic sports. He's trained athletes to compete in four Olympic Games, two Commonwealth Games, and numerous World and European championships. More recently, he's turned his attention to professional golf and football. No one knows better than Nick that training is about results, and this book will help you get them.

High-performance athletes and teams seek out Nick to take them to new heights, and Nick is an expert you should listen to – not because he works with high-profile athletes and teams, but because alongside his coaching commitments with high-performance athletes, he has managed to work with real people in the real world. What many people don't know is that, throughout his career, Nick has always continued to work with normal people on an everyday basis, bringing to the general public his unique combination of fundamental principles and innovative ideas, allowing everyone to train like an athlete.

Each chapter of this book will have been researched, applied and observed in the real world so that the training guidelines that Nick shares with you can be applied to beginners and advanced trainees alike. Although the information in this book is normally only shared with high-performance athletes and coaches, Nick has managed, in his own inimitable style, to make the complex seem simple and the difficult achievable, providing you with an easy-to-understand and logical training system. His book will help any competitive or recreational athlete, as well as those who simply want to unlock their athletic potential.

This book will teach you the fundamentals of training without the need for hype!

Welcome to Nick's world – where everyone can train like an athlete.

Adam Beard MSc, ASCC
Director of High Performance - Cleveland Browns
Head of Physical Performance - Welsh Rugby Union - 2009-2015
Head of Fitness - 2013 British & Irish Lions Tour
UKSCA Strength and Conditioning Coach of the Year 2013

PREFACE

■ **What can you do** to improve your current fitness levels? How can you make sure you don't pull a hamstring playing football? What's the most effective training method to improve your 10km time? What do you need to do to make sure you can keep up with your grandchildren?

Sure, you can train harder, spend more hours at the gym, pound the streets for hours on end in an attempt to eke out some extra improvements in your performance. But wouldn't you rather train a bit smarter, rather than harder?

Ask yourself two important questions

1. **Do you want** to improve your fitness training so that you are in the best shape of your life and you have the confidence that your body can do what you want it to?

2. **If I told you** that there are some simple strategies that can help you optimise your training and performance, would you use them?

What were your answers?

If you answered yes to both questions, read on, because in this book I'm going to explain how a well-designed integrated performance conditioning (IPC) programme can help you achieve your personal fitness goals. I'm going to show you how to 'train like an athlete'. The good news is that you don't need to quit your job and turn pro! Simply read this book to discover how the pros do it.

If you answered no to either of the questions, then you can stop reading now and go and do something else, safe in the knowledge that your fitness goals will always remain just out of reach!

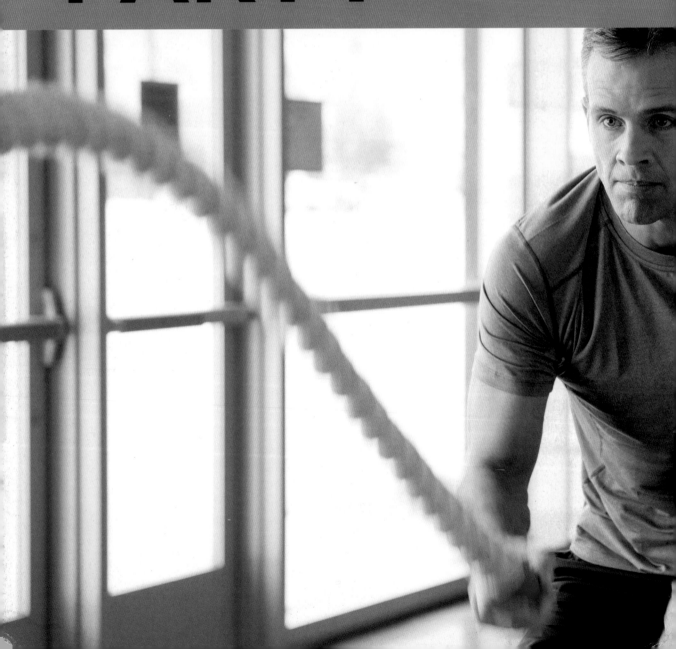

PART I

TRAINING CONCEPTS

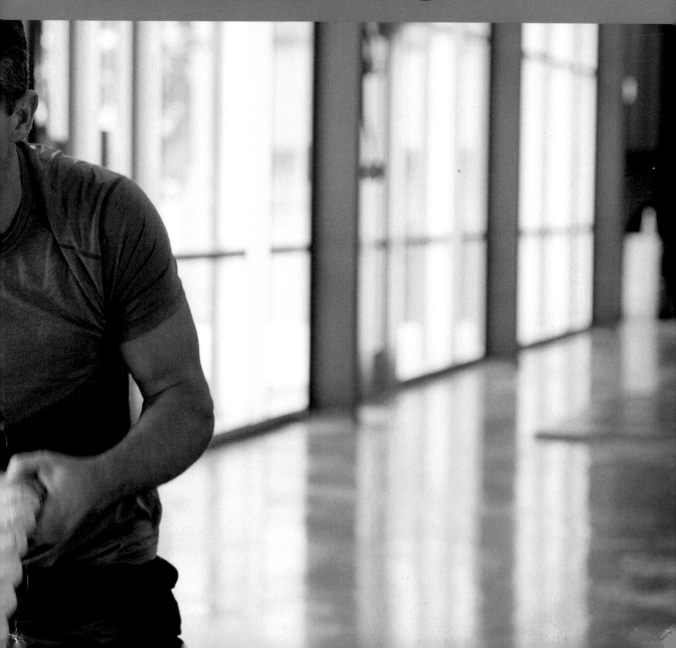

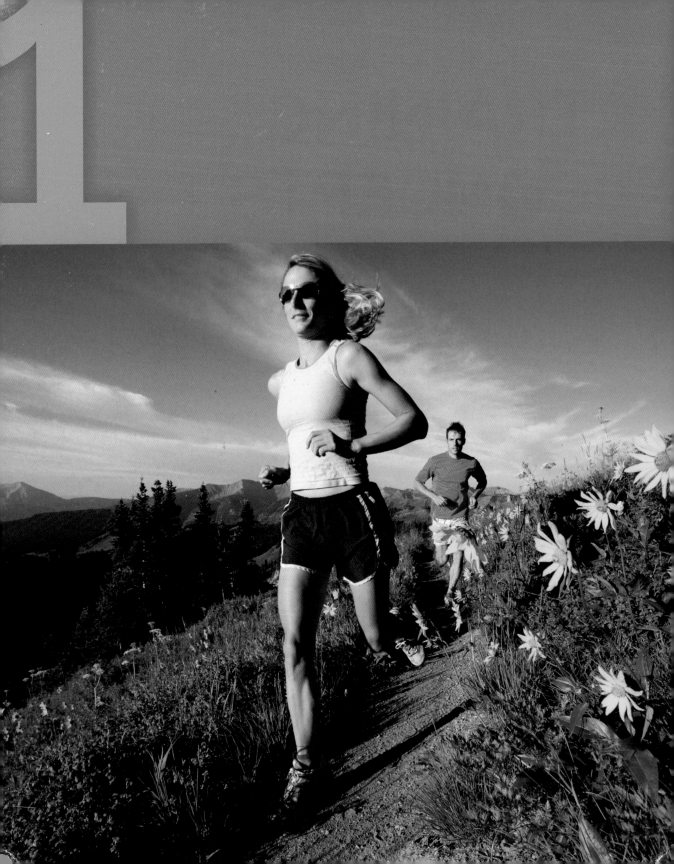

INTRODUCTION: THE ROLE OF S&C IN BEING THE BEST YOU CAN BE

■ **The human body was designed to function** as an integrated unit, so why do so many mainstream training programmes fail to develop total-body functional fitness?

Is *The Strength & Conditioning Bible: How to Train Like an Athlete* really appropriate for you? Absolutely. Most fitness enthusiasts' and recreational athletes' training is ineffective, based on outdated information, old wives' tales and hearsay. It would seem that pretty much everyone thinks they are an expert in this area, and are often more than willing to offer their opinion on how you should be training. Simply mention that you've joined a gym or are training for a marathon and sit back while friends, family and colleagues offer you their pearls of wisdom on precisely the best way to get fit, usually preceded by the words 'when I trained for…'. As well-meaning as this advice is, why would you trust your next-door neighbour (who, after all, spends all day working in IT for a living) with your health and well-being? This is your body we are talking about. You only get given one, so surely you want to ensure that what you do to it is based on something a little more robust than what your neighbour (remember they work in IT all day!) picked up from a magazine they read in the dentist's waiting room!

You can listen to the advice offered by your next-door neighbour, or you can read this book and access the combined knowledge and experience of a coach (that's me, by the way) who has forged a successful career from developing highly effective training programmes for some of the country's most successful athletes. I've been working in high-performance sport for more than 15 years and I've figured out that the secret to success is to develop integrated conditioning programmes that are efficient and effective, and will optimise training results to ensure that the work taking place in the gym impacts directly on performance. I've used these tried-and-tested training methods in high-performance sport and I've also successfully implemented my training strategies with recreational athletes, weekend warriors and the general population. If your training goal is to either improve your athletic performance or get into the best shape of your life, you cannot underestimate the value of integrated performance conditioning and the impact it will have on your performance.

Professional athletes' careers and livelihoods depend on results, so when they turn up to train they make sure they get the most out of every session. You are no different. I've worked with athletes from 35 different sports and not only have they been at the peak of their athletic ability, they have had bodies that could grace the front cover of any health and fitness magazine. Believe me when I tell you that you don't get into that sort of shape following traditional bodybuilding programmes; it's purely a side effect of no-nonsense integrated performance conditioning programmes.

In this book I'm going to introduce you to integrated performance conditioning (IPC). I'm going to share with you the training strategies and principles used by elite athletes and show you how, regardless of your current fitness level and exercise experience, 'anyone can train like an athlete'. I think that last line is worth repeating.

> ## Anyone can train like an athlete

The detailed information in this book will provide a sound scientific rationale for an athletic approach to training and will address key elements of an IPC programme, explaining why adopting a more athletic-based approach to your training will be far superior to what's

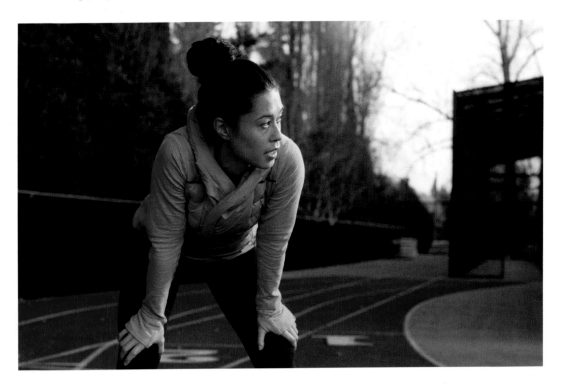

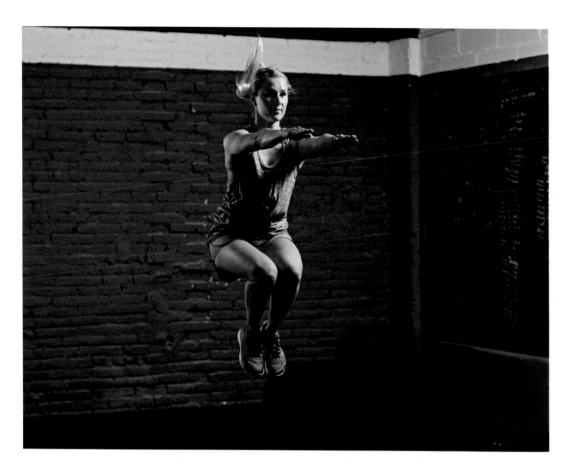

currently on offer to you in the mainstream. You are going to develop a better understanding of physical preparation and you'll be armed with the tools that will enable you to elevate your outdated training programmes and performances to a new level.

A well-designed strength and IPC programme will help you unlock your potential. In the final section of the book you'll find a 16-week, four-stage plan that balances total-body strength, endurance, mobility, balance, coordination and athleticism, and you will be able to develop customisable and realistic fitness programmes. While you are likely to find this programme more challenging than traditional ones that you have followed, the upside is that you will experience greater gains in less time and using less equipment. You are going to realise that you no longer need to spend hours in the gym mindlessly moving from machine to machine. All you need is a maximum of 60 minutes, some space, and simple equipment.

The knowledge gleaned from this book will allow you to develop and enjoy productive and pain-free workouts for many years to come. This book is for you!

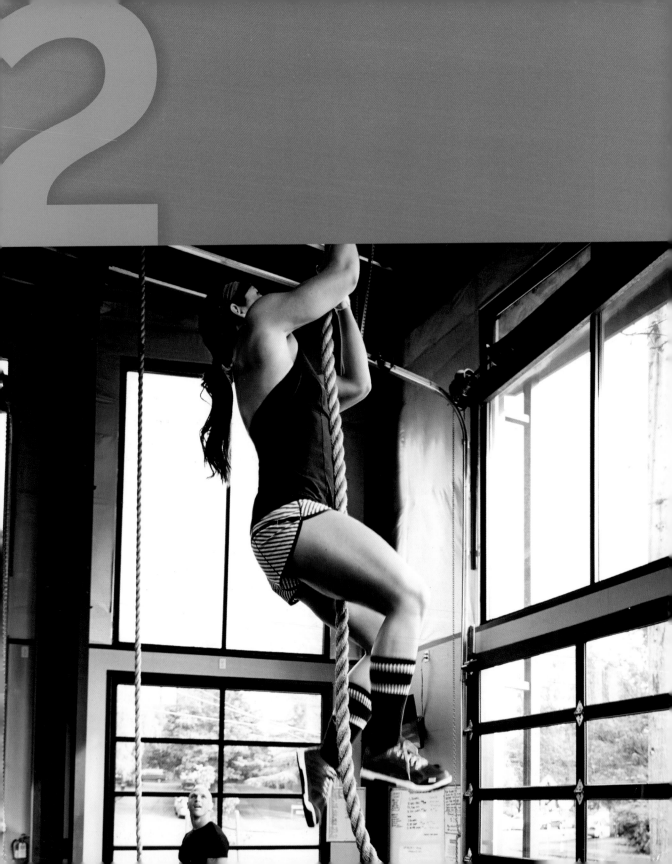

WHAT IS INTEGRATED PERFORMANCE CONDITIONING (IPC)?

■ **Anyone can 'work hard',** it's easy to 'empty the tanks'. The difficult thing for you to do is to ensure that your training sessions are productive and have a purpose. IPC is simply a 'real-world' approach to training and if you look at what each word means you can quickly figure out what IPC sets out to achieve.

Integrated (adjective)	**Performance (noun)**	**Conditioning (noun)**
– with various parts or aspects linked or coordinated	– the action or process of performing a task or function	– bring (something) into the desired state for use

❝*Strength and conditioning covers a wide range of areas that need to be integrated effectively to bring about a performance outcome.*❞

Duncan French PhD, ASCC, CSCS, ASCA-L2. Technical Lead for Strength & Conditioning, English Institute of Sport

Integrated

Possibly the single most important component of this training philosophy is that every element of training is linked and coordinated with a view to improving performance. Traditionally, fitness coaches and athletes have adopted a unimodal approach to training, primarily focusing on the development of one fitness component at the expense of others. Let's say you wanted to get fit so that you could run a local 10km race. The logical starting point for most people would be to spend hours clocking up miles running out on the streets in an attempt to develop lungs like dustbin liners and a body that could withstand the constant pounding that running inflicts on the body! Certainly this is a tried-and-tested option, but is it the most efficient and effective approach? What other fitness components would help improve performance? Could they be integrated into your training programme to boost performance?

Modern training science has shown us that the more effective way to improve performance is to adopt an integrated approach. How does this work in reality? Using the earlier example of getting fit for a local 10km race, several fitness components should be integrated into the training programme to ensure it's as effective as possible. If I were writing the programme, I would integrate the following components:

Strength

The ability to control and produce force is an important component of running performance. Increased strength levels will improve running economy, making life on the streets much easier. Increased strength levels will also help reduce injury potential.

Injury Reduction

The highly repetitive nature of running and the impact on the body can often result in chronic overuse injuries. Applying some simple remedial conditioning exercises to build in 'functional capacity' would help to reduce the number and severity of running-based injuries.

Recovery and Regeneration

Often neglected, but a cornerstone of every good training programme, an effective recovery strategy can make all the difference to fitness gains and performances.

As you can see from the example, simply running to get fit for running is not the most effective and efficient way of doing things. Integrating three complementary fitness components will ultimately bring about greater gains in fitness and performance. By adopting an integrated approach to conditioning, you can develop your ability to work to a higher level with less energy cost, improving efficiency and economy of movement (metabolic and mechanical).

'Understanding the different contributing factors to performance and improvement allow you to make your own informed decisions later on around exercise choice, recovery and elements of programming.'
Pete McKnight BSc, CSCS, ASCC. Chairman of the UKSCA Strength & Conditioning Coach, French Ski Team

Performance

Inspired by the famous Penrose Steps (also known as the Impossible Staircase, an optical illusion that depicts people walking round a series of steps that inevitably brings them back to the same place), what I often witness in training venues around the world is the 'march of futility'. People working out but never getting anywhere, ending up back at the beginning, where the whole journey starts again. If you don't have a training plan linked to a performance outcome then there is no plan to your training and you are ultimately just 'doing work', treading the same path but always returning to the same point. It is important to remember that all training needs to have a purpose, over and above 'emptying the tanks'.

Making people work is easy. I can 'empty' anyone in the space of a few minutes, I can probably make them sick and I'll make them so sore they'll have to stay in bed for a week, but is that going to help the athlete achieve their performance outcome? The goal of every training session is to bring about an adaptive response (being sick is a response but not really one we should be chasing!). Lots of you reading this book will love to train but are probably simply putting the hours in, without much consideration of what you actually want to achieve. Unfortunately, lots of coaches are doing exactly the same when they put together your training programmes! For training to be effective it has to be related to the task or performance outcome. When I spoke to renowned strength and conditioning coach Vern Gambetta, he simply said 'everyone should train with a purpose'.

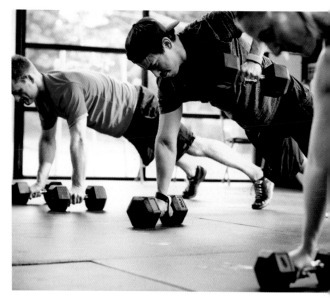

△ Train with a purpose

> ❛*The greatest question you can ask yourself while training is "why"? "Why am I doing this and why now?" If your goal is clear and compelling enough you will easily answer the "why" question. If your goal is clear and the activity doesn't help you to achieve it then change the activity.*❜
>
> **Richard Nugent** M.D. TwentyOne Leadership and Success In Football

It's important that you realise that your training must be linked to the end goal. It needs to be functional (I'll explain exactly what this means in more detail later in this section) but basically all movements have a level of functionality, and if training moves too far away from fundamental movements it will be less effective. If you want to be able to play five-a-side football with your friends, your training must be 'task orientated'. Five-a-side football can be physically demanding, with lots of changes of direction, sudden bursts of speed, body contact etc. If this is your performance outcome, you need to make sure that the exercises you are performing in your training sessions are preparing you for the demands of the game. In my experience, most five-a-side enthusiasts are poorly prepared (just look at the number of players who hobble home with an injury at the end of a game).

Conditioning

'Conditioning' can take on different meanings, but I like the dictionary term used earlier in this section, 'bring (something) into the desired state for use'.

For me, conditioning is all about developing the 'functional capacity' needed to improve and deliver performance, and that doesn't happen overnight. It takes time and effort to ensure that your body is capable of doing what you want it to do without breaking down. Those final three words are worth reiterating: without breaking down. We are probably all capable of producing a one-off performance, be it a game of football with our kids, a quick sprint across the road or a marathon to raise money for charity. But at what cost does that performance come and can we repeat it again and again? I've seen professional athletes, weekend warriors and newbie marathon runners who can all produce one or even a handful of performances, but who ultimately break down due to a lack of functional capacity because they've not taken the time to develop an appropriate level of underpinning conditioning.

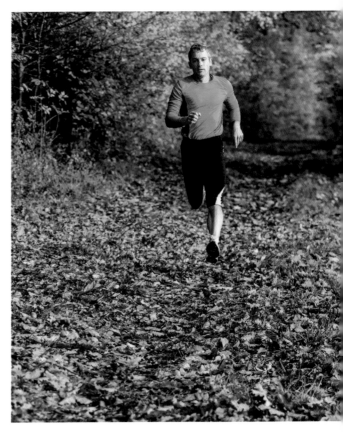

△ 'Get fit' to cope with the demands of the activity

> If you want your body to perform a task (kick a ball, run for the bus, lift up your grandchildren, run a marathon) and, more importantly, if you want to be able to repeat that task without the fear of injury, your body must have an appropriate level of conditioning to cope with the demands being placed upon it.

❝Don't just think of conditioning for your specific sport ... otherwise you will be seeking regular medical attention!! Read on...❞

Grant Downie OBE. MCSP HCPC. Head of Performance, Manchester City FC Academy

A classic mistake that is often made, and one that I see happening time and time again, is when someone decides to take up a sport in an attempt to 'get fit'. Filled with good intentions, they traipse off to the local ... (insert sport of your choice, anything from triathlon or marathon-running to mixed martial arts, etc) and dive head first into some very specific and surprisingly demanding training. Unable to walk properly the next day, they realise that this is absolutely the wrong approach to getting back into shape! The first step should always be to 'get fit' to cope with the demands of the activity you would like to take part in. If you want to take up a new sport or you're already out there taking part in recreational sport, you need to ask yourself: 'Do I have the "functional capacity"' needed to improve and deliver performance or am I just one session or game away from an injury?' Your training programme should develop your ability to tolerate workloads and to resist and recover from fatigue.

Components of Integrated Performance Conditioning

'*Resistance training and running/cardio is not a fitness program. It's a piece of a programme.*

A complete programme needs movement skills, power, elasticity, core stability work, "corrective" work, alongside resistance training and energy system work. And then you need to recover and regenerate from the work in that programme. It has to all fit.

It's like an artist having different colours on their paint palette. Mix them well and you can create a masterpiece. Dump them all together without thought and you just end up with a mess.'

Alwyn Cosgrove. Owner, Results Fitness

The first step you need to take in order to train like a modern-day athlete is to recognise that a fundamental shift in your mindset is required if you are to develop a comprehensive physical preparation programme that delivers optimal levels of fitness and function. If endurance is your thing, simply grinding out more endurance efforts isn't going to cut it; you need to think about movement quality training,

strength and power development and injury reduction strategies. If you are a busy parent juggling the demands of home, children, work and sport, you need to think about doing less, improving your training density and focusing on recovery and regeneration strategies. You need to open yourself up to the potential that an IPC programme has to offer. Step outside of your box and get ready to train for the demands of the 'real world'.

A well-developed IPC programme will incorporate elements from these six key training areas:

1. Movement Quality Training (MQT)
2. Flexibility and Mobility
3. Strength and Power
4. Injury Reduction and Rehabilitation
5. Metabolic Conditioning
6. Recovery and Regeneration.

1. MOVEMENT QUALITY TRAINING (MQT)

Development of gross athleticism and coordinated skilful movements.

The starting point for an IPC programme is to develop gross athleticism through MQT so that you can produce coordinated and skilful movements. Your body needs to be able to perform a wide and varied range of activities. You need the body to be able to function as a whole. The programmes that have been developed for this book will probably look completely different to the typical one that you have followed in the past, and here's why. We all share common movement patterns that need to be developed – squat, hinge, pull (vertical and horizontal), push (vertical and horizontal), lunge, carry, reach, lift, accelerate, and decelerate – but most programmes fall well short of the mark when it comes to improving movement quality. Can you stand on one leg for 60 seconds without falling over? Does your squat resemble a curtsy to the Queen or can you perform a full-range squat with flawless technique?

Let's think about movement in terms of vocabulary (a set of words that are familiar to you). Your vocabulary usually develops as you get older, and is a fundamental tool for communication. If you have a limited vocabulary, it's going to be pretty tough for you to communicate effectively. Just look at an 18-month-old baby trying to tell you they are hungry – chances are you have no idea what they are asking for, it could be anything from food, a clean nappy, sleep etc etc! Acquiring an extensive vocabulary is a challenge but it is fundamental to effective communication. The building blocks of vocabulary are words and the building blocks of words are the letters of the alphabet. We need to understand the alphabet to build words and develop an extensive vocabulary.

Movement is something that should also develop and improve as we get older. As we grow we learn to roll, crawl, sit, stand, hop, skip, jump, walk and run, and these fundamental movements are the movement equivalent of the letters of the alphabet. If we have good fundamental movement patterns (letters of the alphabet), we can link them together to produce more complex and challenging movements (words) and develop an extensive 'movement vocabulary' that we can use in day-to-day and sporting activities.

The most successful athletes are the ones with the largest movement vocabulary. If you only have movements A–D, your movement vocabulary is going to be pretty limited. The problem faced by many of you will be that, over time, you've probably done a pretty amazing job of forgetting how to move efficiently and effectively. Far from improving with age, movement often deteriorates as you get older through a combination of factors: lifestyle, work, sedentary living, injury and illness. Trying to perform complex movements with a limited movement vocabulary sets you up for problems further down the line.

Your body is a highly complex organism and MQT is designed to reinforce the correct postures and positions of the body during movement in order to allow for effective transfer and expression of force and power. If you want to be capable of delivering fluid, athletic movements, you need to spend time on MQT and develop your gross athleticism.

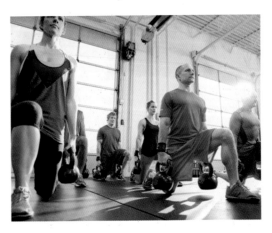

◁ Develop an extensive movement vocabulary

> *Winning in elite sport frequently depends on getting positive outcomes from calculated risks. From the physical perspective, the better your performance programme is the more accurate your calculations become.*

Dr Mark Gillett MSc (SEM) FRCS FCEM(UK&I) Dip IMC RCSEd. Director of Performance, West Bromwich Albion FC

2. FLEXIBILITY AND MOBILITY

Increasing joint range of motion (ROM) using a range of strategies (soft tissue work, self-myofascial release, static stretching, neuromuscular, dynamic and strength).

Flexibility and mobility training is possibly the most forgotten, misunderstood and misapplied aspect of physical preparation and it's probably the first part of training to get dropped when time is tight. There are many different training approaches available and later on in the book we will discuss in detail the various types of flexibility and mobility exercises and how they can be integrated effectively to increase functional range of motion. Take on a multi-modal approach but remember, the key is to avoid a 'stretch everything' mentality; prioritise the areas that need the most work and integrate a range of complementary techniques to increase functional range of motion. Working to improve flexibility is time well spent; it will allow you to move easily through an unrestricted, pain-free range of motion and that will definitely improve your training and competition performances.

> *Limits in functional flexibility can significantly impair the ability to move efficiently.*

Gambetta, 2007

3. STRENGTH AND POWER

Use of a range of training methods to develop sub-qualities of strength (conditioning, hypertrophy, maximum strength, power, reactive strength, strength endurance).

The human body has over 660 muscles (40–45 per cent of its total mass), which when combined with other connective tissues transmit force to the skeletal system to produce movement (Cardinale, Newton & Nosaka, 2011). Strength gains are due to: 1) neuromuscular adaptations, 2) increased cross-sectional area (CSA) or 3) a combination of both. Strength and power training causes adaptive changes on various systems within the body, including the musculoskeletal system (structure and architecture of skeletal muscle, tendons), the neuromuscular system (contractile rate) and neuroendocrine system (regulation of protein synthesis and muscle growth).

Strength and power training ultimately leads to improved mechanical muscle function, which in turn results in improved functional performance in various activities of day-to-day life, including: athletic performance, general health, rehabilitation and reconditioning, counteraction of aging-induced muscle loss. But not everyone reading this book will be convinced that strength and power development can help their training. Let's take the recreational endurance athlete as an example. How can strength and power training possibly help them? When working with endurance athletes, they will often ask, 'Why do I need to work on improving my strength?' You may think it's a fair question; after all, for most endurance athletes the benefits of strength training are outweighed by the fear of gaining too much bulk, loss of flexibility and diminished 'feel' of their sport. But let's get one thing clear right now: strength training for endurance athletes is not about developing a 'beach body' or turning them into a muscle-bound hulk. I've worked with enough athletes to know that a good strength-training programme will not only make them stronger, faster and more economical but will help them to remain injury free.

Benefits of Strength and Power Development

- Increased strength and power
- Improved neural functioning
- Increased rate of force development (RFD)
- Improved fine motor control
- Structural modifications in bone
- Improved tendon CSA and morphology
- Adaptive responses in testosterone, cortisol and growth hormone

4. INJURY REDUCTION AND REHABILITATION

Integrated corrective strategies to address movement deficiencies and injuries.

How many times have you continued to train around a pre-existing problem? Think about all of the times you played rugby with a sore knee or went for another swim knowing that at the end of the session your shoulder was going to be throbbing. How many times have you seen a physiotherapist who has identified a weakness or muscle imbalance that you need to work on, only to subsequently ignore their advice? How long did you stick to the rehabilitation programme? Do you actually train your weaknesses?

If you love sport, the chances are you'll have picked up an injury at some point and here's the problem.

> Previous injury associated with inadequate rehabilitation predisposes you to recurrence of further injury.

I work with injured athletes on a daily basis and I can tell you that injuries ruin motivation and can have a significant impact on the athletes' ability to perform at their best. The same applies to you. It's obvious, really – if you aren't healthy, you can't train to the best of your ability, and progress will be limited. If you've not incorporated injury reduction strategies into your programme, you're setting yourself up for a fall – it's just around the corner, and when it hits you, you'll be wondering why you sat back and did nothing about it before it struck. Putting in place a solid injury reduction and reconditioning programme will be a major factor in the success of your programme and that's why it is one of the six key components of IPC.

5. METABOLIC CONDITIONING

Developing the ability to tolerate workloads and produce effort with minimal decrement.

Metabolic conditioning is a term used to describe conditioning exercises intended to increase the storage and delivery of energy for any activity. The term metabolic system refers to three distinct yet closely related integrated processes:

- Splitting of the stored phosphagens – ATP-PC System (immediate)
- Anaerobic breakdown of carbohydrate – Anaerobic System (short)
- Aerobic breakdown of carbohydrates and fats – Aerobic System (long)

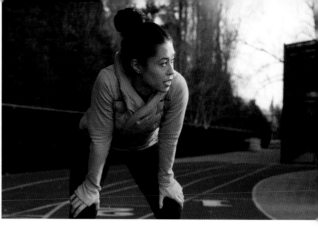

△ You need to plan 'time outs'

Your IPC programme should develop the appropriate metabolic system. The real goal for the majority of you will be to develop a strong foundation of general fitness 'work capacity' – the ability to tolerate a workload and recover from it.

6. RECOVERY AND REGENERATION

Fundamental for optimal adaptation-reduced risk of injury and illness.

For years, recovery and regeneration has been hidden in the shadows, eclipsed by fitness training, but in recent years our understanding of fatigue and its impact on performance means that recovery and regeneration is now at the forefront of advances in programme design.

In order for the body to be able to adapt to training, it must have a period of sufficient recovery. This is not a new concept – Hans Selye first proposed it back in the 1940s and it should be one of the cornerstones of your training programme.

Your body is pretty amazing and actually needs a certain level of physiological stress to bring about physiological adaptations, which ultimately lead to improved performances.

Training creates that physiological stress; it disturbs homeostasis at a cellular level. This is just what the body ordered, but only if you allow some time for it to recover.

Recovery provides an opportunity for training-based adaptations to take place, enabling the body to cope with the subsequent training session. To encourage adaptation to training, it is important to plan recovery activities that reduce residual fatigue. That's right, you need to plan 'time outs' because without sufficient rest your body cannot adapt to and cope with the physical and mental demands of training and it will fairly quickly become exhausted.

IPC isn't a fad, it's not the latest training concept, it is simply a 'real-world' approach to training that draws on fundamental training principles to establish a logical and systematic approach to training.

'*Every S&C coach needs to be able to work with specialists in other areas like medical, nutrition and technical coaches to guide desired outcomes.*'

Darren Roberts High Performance Manager, Harris and Ross Healthcare

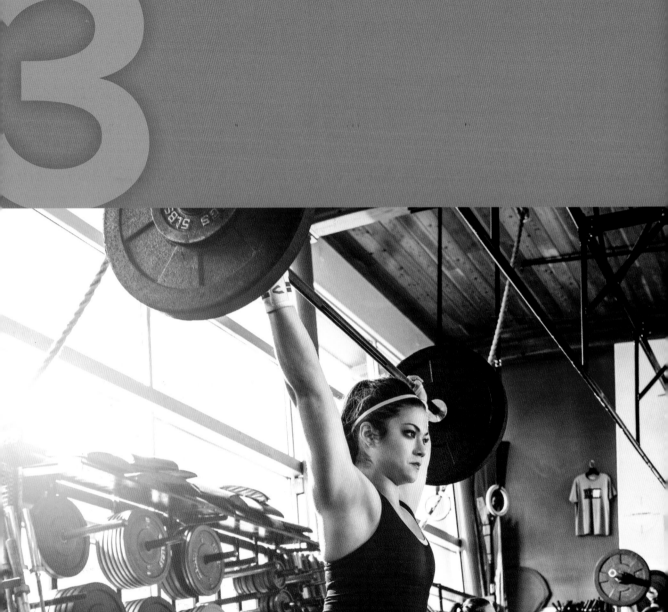

FIVE-POINT BLUEPRINT FOR SUCCESS

■ **Five key training concepts provide the foundations** on which to develop an effective IPC programme. These are the cornerstones of my training philosophy and when I'm asked to work with an athlete or team they are the fundamental principles that I always come back to.

They've worked for me throughout my career and if you keep them at the forefront of your mind when developing your personal IPC programme, I know that they will help you achieve your performance outcome.

'*The most effective plan will always be the simplest.*'

Duncan French PhD, ASCC, CSCS, ASCA-L2. Technical Lead for Strength & Conditioning, English Institute of Sport

Quality

> **Develop a set of fundamental movement skills that focus on quality of movement before quantity.**

Your primary goal when you want to improve your training is to establish technical competency in fundamental movement patterns and that can only be achieved by consistently and rigorously maintaining the quality of what you do.

One of the challenges I constantly face is to convince the athletes and coaches that I work with to chase quality of movement before quantity. I don't really care how much work you can do, I care about the quality of the work being produced.

We've already discussed how easy it is to simply 'work'. The trick is to make sure that everything you do is of the highest possible quality. Of course, your technique isn't always going to be flawless, particularly when learning new movements or when you're fatigued. But the minute you accept poor-quality movement that is outside the 'buffer' of acceptable technique in favour of quantity is the moment you accept substandard performances and increased injury potential.

A couple of classic examples are:

The guy in the squat rack at the gym with a fully loaded bar busting out squats with a rounded back and knees that look like they are trying to kiss each other. This is a classic case of accepting quantity (hitting big numbers on the bar) over quality (ensuring technique is flawless and range of motion is optimal). If that were my athlete, we would be stripping the bar down to a weight that they could lift while maintaining acceptable technique. Ego gets parked at the door!

The cyclist who goes out for a long ride but bimbles along at a pace that an asthmatic octogenarian could keep up with. Yes, they can update their social media profile and tell their cycling buddies that they've been in the saddle for 4 hours but they've gone big on quantity at the expense of quality. If that were my athlete, we would be looking at putting together a training ride that relied less on time in the saddle (a results by volume approach) and more on quality and training intensity.

Functional

Achieving pain-free movement patterns and developing function for daily activity while avoiding injury should be primary objectives of any training programme. The human body is complex and fitness training must take into account how the musculoskeletal system actually functions and at the same time consider the physiological adaptations that we are trying to bring about. Multi-joint exercises using multiple muscle groups will recruit considerably more muscle mass than a single joint or machine variation. Real-world activities require all of your muscles to work at the same time and, as discussed earlier in this section, it is important that you should 'learn the alphabet' and develop gross athleticism and coordinated skilful movements.

Functional training typically progresses from general training to more specific training, developing the ability to perform integrated multi-dimensional movements at various loads and speeds. Often you will need to 'get fit' to cope with the amount of training needed to improve performance and, during the initial stage of training, programmes should develop your ability to tolerate workloads and to resist and recover from fatigue.

While all movements have a level of functionality, it is vital that you understand that the level of functionality is related to the performance outcome you want to achieve. Consider every exercise and training session in relation to the outcome.

'*If training moves too far away from fundamental movements there will be less transfer of training effect [degree to which a training exercise as part of a programme affects the long-term performance improvement].*'
Gambetta, 2007

A comprehensive training programme will incorporate training methods and techniques

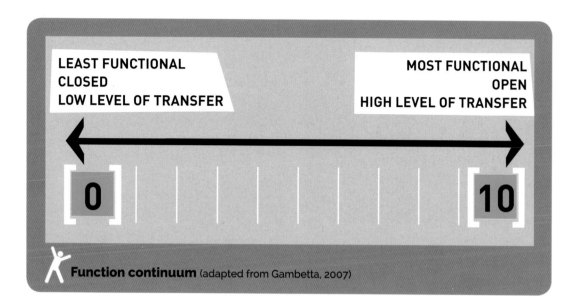

LEAST FUNCTIONAL
CLOSED
LOW LEVEL OF TRANSFER

MOST FUNCTIONAL
OPEN
HIGH LEVEL OF TRANSFER

0   10

Function continuum (adapted from Gambetta, 2007)

that span the continuum, with a greater emphasis towards the right-hand side (bodyweight, freeweight, ground-based and compound movements). That's not to say that you should never include exercises toward the left-hand side of the continuum (isolation exercises, machine-based), they just have to have an impact on your performance outcome. Once you have developed the capacity to tolerate training and have established the ability to perform integrated multi-dimensional movements at various loads and speeds, you can start to develop the ability to produce high levels of work with minimal fatigue. At this point, programmes should be directed towards higher-intensity workloads with an 'athletic' expression of strength.

When selecting a training intervention, consider the following factors and the impact they will have on the functional nature of the exercise. This bit gets a little 'sciency' but I'll try to keep it brief!

‘*Success will be achieved when the art of coaching flows seamlessly with the underpinning science necessary to fully understand the athlete and the sport.*’

Neil Parsley BSc, CSCS, ASCC. Director, Underground Training Station

KINEMATICS – WHAT DOES THE MOVEMENT ACTUALLY LOOK LIKE?

Kinematics is the study of motion without taking into account forces that cause it.
The basic movements of the human body can be described in terms of planes of motion (sagittal – divides the body into right and left; frontal – divides the body into front and back; transverse – divides the body into top and bottom), number of joints, speed of movement, and the range and direction of the movement.

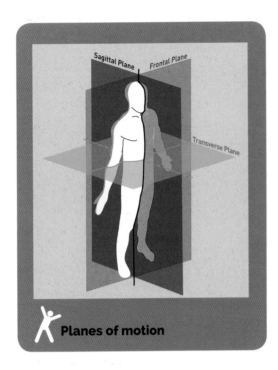

Planes of motion

KINETICS – WHAT CAUSES MOVEMENT?

Kinetics is concerned with the forces involved to actually bring about movement.
This is a critical component of functional training but is often overlooked for the more obvious 'movement – kinematic' approach to exercise selection, i.e. if it looks like the sports movement then it must be a good exercise. Kinematics is really important because even if the exercise looks good, the way it is performed (speed of movement, ranges at which force is produced, how quickly force is produced and the time it takes to generate maximum force) could be completely inappropriate for the performance outcome.

Integral to exercise selection is an understanding of the force velocity curve and the impact that has on the training outcome and functionality of the exercise.

We will look at the various strength qualities in more depth later on in the book but you can see from the force velocity curve that we can develop different types of strength. For example, if I want to improve maximum strength I'll need to move a big heavy load (produce lots of force) and that load won't move very quickly (slow velocity). If I decided that I needed to improve my reactive strength then I would work at the opposite end of the force velocity curve and try to move lighter loads (typically bodyweight) as quickly as possible (fast velocity).

Endurance athletes often base a lot of their training slap bang in the middle of the force velocity curve, choosing to focus on sessions in the gym that develop strength endurance. It makes logical sense, right? Endurance runners need good strength endurance, therefore let's perform circuit training with moderate loads and high repetitions. This may be appropriate for some endurance athletes but potential

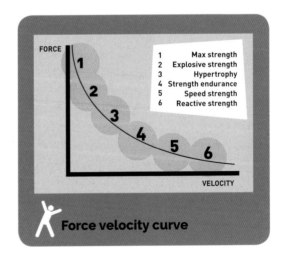

Force velocity curve

gains at opposite ends of the force velocity curve (maximum strength or reactive strength) may actually provide a bigger return.

> To select the most appropriate exercise and ensure that it's completed with the correct kinematics, we need to understand what strength qualities we already posses and how these need to be developed in order to improve performance.

ENERGETICS

When muscles work, they require energy so that they can contract. Chemical energy is transformed into mechanical energy and that results in movement (OK, it's a little bit more complicated in reality but that's essentially it). We have three different metabolic systems at our disposal to produce chemical energy:

- **ATP-PC** – provides instant energy but once that supply has been exhausted (potential for 5–10 seconds of energy supply), the body will need to find anther way to produce energy.
- **Anaerobic** – capable of producing energy rapidly for large (high-intensity) but short-term power outputs (potential for another 60–120 seconds of energy supply).
- **Aerobic** – produces energy at a slower rate for low–moderate intensity and long duration activities (potential to supply energy for up to 2 hours of activity).

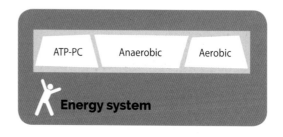

We will look at the energy systems in more detail later on in the book, but when discussing energetics in relation to the selection of functional training activities we must recognise that the contribution from each energy system varies according to the intensity and duration of the activity and the body's fuel supply.

You need to consider the total duration of the activity you are training for as well as the typical time frames for efforts within that activity. Old-school thinking would have you believe that football players need to be able to run for 90 minutes, which is why back in the day it wouldn't have been unusual to see football players heading out for a long run as part of their physical preparation (they used to think sucking on an orange segment at half time was a good idea, too!). Our understanding of the game is much more advanced now and while players *are* on the pitch for 90 minutes, they are not running around at a steady pace; in fact, a lot of their efforts will be high-tempo with periods of rest in between. Training needs to reflect the demands of the sport and careful selection of training sessions is key to the development of the appropriate energy supply systems.

Functional training is not about circus tricks. Functional means using the most appropriate training methods to enhance your performance. The key to success is selecting exercises that will maximise the transfer of training effect to ensure that what you do in the gym impacts directly on performance. The more boxes an exercise ticks (kinematics, kinetics, energetics), the more functional it is.

Efficient

Why would you want to spend any more time than was absolutely necessary working out in the gym or pounding the streets in preparation for a half-marathon? Yes, you read that right, the fitness expert has just asked you why you would want to be training any longer than you needed to be! I'm not giving you permission to kick back, relax and let your body drift slowly into a state of decline. I'm telling you that, while fitness training is important, you need to 'train like an athlete' and make sure that your time spent working out is efficient and effective. Later on in the book I'll show you how to develop training programmes that can deliver great results without you having to make the gym your second home; but for now I'm going to share with you one habit you can adopt from professional athletes that will improve your training efficiency.

We live in a 24-hour society and demands on our time seem to be constantly increasing. It's tough to maintain a structured training programme when you are a professional athlete; it's even harder when you are trying to juggle the demands of a full-time job, young family, hectic social life or possibly all three. Professional athletes' careers and livelihoods depend on results, so when they turn up to train they make sure they get the most out

of every session. They don't simply turn up to training and go through the motions. To ensure every session is as time-efficient as possible, they train with 'intent'.

> **Intent (adjective)** – having the will and mind focused on a specific purpose

I've worked with hundreds of recreational athletes and weekend warriors who are training really really hard (I know this because they tell everyone via various social media platforms that they've just trained really really hard!) and getting nowhere. They are simply spinning their wheels, spending hours in the gym or pounding the streets with nothing more to show for their efforts than a badge of honour that says 'I trained six times this week'. They are not training with intent, they are not getting the most out of every session.

Are you training with intent? Here's a clue: if you can read a magazine while on the bike in the gym, compile your shopping list during a spin class or catch a glimpse of your favourite soap on the TV while performing lunges, you're not training with intent. If you don't find yourself chatting to people between sets in the gym, if you can only think about your lungs bursting as you step up the pace on your final mile or the fact that your knee alignment during your squat needs to be better, you're training with intent!

Exercise selection and programme design have a significant impact on the duration of a training session but *you* can also have a direct impact on the efficiency and effectiveness of your training session. Time is a non-renewable resource; don't waste it by training ineffectively. Training like an athlete means having a programme that uses the minimum 'dose' but delivers the maximum 'effect'. It also means making sure you focus during the session on a specific outcome and train with intent.

> **A 'results by volume' approach to training is inefficient.**

Continuity

Why do most people fail to hit their performance outcome? Lack of continuity in their training. It seems that most people are incapable of sticking to a plan and prefer to 'freestyle' their training. There are two components to continuity that will ensure success: 1) how often you train, and 2) how much variety you have in your training.

Training continuity is like depositing money into a bank account. If I deposit £10 every day for 60 days, I'll have £600 in my account. If, however, I'm a bit hit and miss and I only manage to get to the bank 25 times during those 60 days to deposit £10, I'll only have £250 in my account. Developing a regular training history (continuity) is going to put 'more money in the bank' and help you develop your fitness 'reserves'. Developing a good 'training history' stands you in good stead for the future when you may need to take some time out, maybe for a holiday or in preparation for a major race. Unlike the person who has only built up 25 days' worth of fitness reserves, you will have

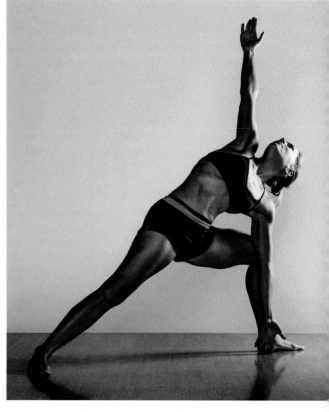

△ Focus during the session on a specific outcome

60 days and can afford to take a bit of time out (take money out of your fitness account without going overdrawn!). The success or failure of your IPC programme will be dependent on your ability to stick to a plan and train consistently over an extended period of time. Three weeks of training is not going to transform you into a champion!

How often should you change your training programme? We live in a world where constant change seems to be seen as a good thing; in fact, there are some training programmes that hold constant change as a cornerstone of training. While doing the same thing over and over again is monotonous and – if you're not seeing results – just plain stupid, too much variety in your training is going to turn you into a jack-of-all-trades but master of none. The time to switch up your programme is when you stop making gains. I'm not suggesting that you just repeat the same old programme year on year, but when it comes to establishing an IPC programme, continuity trumps variety every time.

Planned variations are essential to elicit training adaptation and your training programmes must be developed with both short- and long-term aims in mind. Random changes in training stimulus every session (putting different amounts of money in the bank account each time) doesn't provide the optimal conditions for physiological adaptation and performance gains.

Training is cumulative and you must develop programmes, not workouts. Always ask the question: 'Why am I changing the programme? Is it because I'm bored, or have I reached a point where I've stopped making gains and need a new stimulus?' If you don't develop a regular training habit and you keep switching from one type of training to another, you will struggle to see improvements in your training and ultimately fail to realise your performance outcomes.

Recovery

If you are reading this book, it's probably because you love to keep fit and want to optimise your training; but how can you push yourself in training without tipping your body over the edge? Training and competing for an event or simply hitting the gym on a regular basis places significant demands on your body. If your ability to recover from training and competition is a limiting factor in your performance, then invisible training (recovery and regeneration) is your secret weapon! Training is designed to progressively overload the body systems and fuel stores and it must be applied carefully to improve performance. Prolonged periods of training with inadequate recovery will dump your body into a hole and a state of fatigue during which training and performance will be compromised.

> Fatigue is multi-factorial and you will experience a number of different forms of fatigue as a result of training and competition: metabolic, tissue damage, neurological, psychological and environmental.

We will take a more detailed look at recovery and regeneration later on in the book, but the main principle to understand is that the ability for your body to regain its physiological balance is dependent on its ability to recover from training and competition. To encourage training adaptations it is important to plan recovery activities that reduce residual fatigue and you should plan periods of recovery and regeneration to provide an opportunity for training-based adaptations to take place. It's easy to get carried away with all the latest fads and trends, such as compression clothing and ice baths, while forgetting about the basics.

Sleep is one of the most important forms of rest and provides time for you to adapt to the physical and mental demands of training. Nutrition (refuelling and rehydration) is also a cornerstone of a comprehensive recovery and regeneration strategy and a solid approach to refuelling and rehydrating will have a positive impact on performance. Body management and the appropriate use of passive and active rest are also beneficial to overall recovery.

Recovery and regeneration is a fundamental component of an IPC programme and if you take the time to put in place some simple recovery and regeneration strategies, you will be able to optimise your training and reduce the risk of injury and illness.

Cornerstones of Physical Preparation

Underpinning the key concepts that we've discussed earlier in this section are six cornerstones of physical preparation. The importance lies in the fact that these are guiding principles backed by science, not a passing fad or bandwagon. In the world of fitness a new training *method* will pop up every 6 months and all across the gyms in the world you will see trainers and their clients abandoning the last big thing to hit the fitness industry in favour of the next big thing! I'm not making this up – in the past decade we've seen everything from kettle-bells, club

swinging, crossfit and suspension training to barefoot running, stability balls and Zumba. The list is endless and so is the turnover.

Athletes and coaches looking for sustained success don't get caught up in training fads. Neither should you. It's not about *methods* or *equipment*; it's about understanding *principles*. Great coaches and athletes will develop programmes based on these cornerstones. Sure, they may use some of the techniques as training tools but they don't base their whole training philosophy on the latest fitness craze.

These are fundamental laws that shape every training decision I make when developing programmes for world-class athletes. These cornerstones are also the bedrock of your training programme, so I think

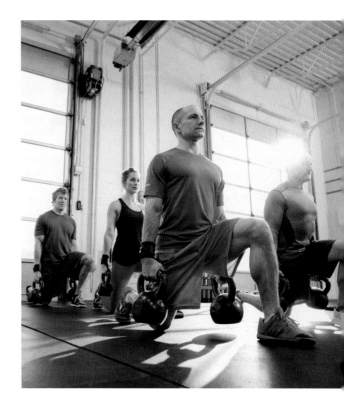

it's important that you become familiar with the strength and conditioning equivalent of the Ten Commandments (but there are only six!).

> *As to methods there may be a million and then some, but principles are few. The man who grasps principles can successfully select his own methods. The man who tries methods, ignoring principles, is sure to have trouble.*
>
> Ralph Waldo Emerson

INDIVIDUAL DIFFERENCES

This is probably the most important cornerstone, that's why it's #1! If you announce to your friend that you are going to tackle a triathlon, you will be offered all sorts of advice. Most of this will be based on your friend's personal experience, or maybe from conversations they've had with fellow competitors at the start line. The advice that is being dished out free of charge by your friend normally has one major issue. Just because the training tip worked for them or a friend of a friend, it doesn't mean it will work for you. Why? Because we are all different. We all have different abilities and weaknesses, and will respond differently (to a degree) to any given stimulus or training system. It sounds so obvious, but it's probably the one thing we always forget when it comes to fitness training. The programme that you need to follow has to work for *you*. Listen to the advice, take on the tips, but make sure it works for you.

ACCOMMODATION

This cornerstone is often brushed over but we have to remember that if we complete the same session (distance covered, weight lifted etc) over and over again, our body will stop responding in the same way. We get used to it. By definition, accommodation is the decrease in response of a biological organism to a continuous stimulus (Zatsiorsky, 1995). If standard training sessions and workloads are used for extended periods of time, inefficiency occurs and the training adaptations that we are chasing will be lost. We know from previous sections that we need continuity in our training – it's part of the five-point blueprint for success – but if left unchecked your fitness levels will start to drop. Being able to correctly choose the optimal progression level for an exercise is an important skill to develop in our training. Your training sessions should always provide you with a challenge.

If you continually choose exercises or loads that are too easy, progress will stall. This is why you will see the same old faces at the gym or passing you on the street while out for a run or bike ride, and they just don't seem to be making any progress. Chances are their sessions haven't changed in months, and neither have their fitness levels. It's

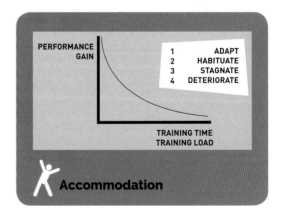

commendable; they are putting the effort in week after week for very little payback. That's not what I want you to be doing. Keep a level of continuity in the programme, but always push yourself a little harder with each new session.

THE GENERAL ADAPTATION SYNDROME (GAS)

The GAS theory was developed by a rather clever chap called Hans Selye back in the 1940s and he established that there must be a period of low-intensity training or complete recovery following periods of intense training. It makes sense, right? Train really hard, put your feet up and have a rest so you are ready for the next session. While it is logical, it's another cornerstone that is often neglected. Recovery from training is important and we've seen from previous sections how it fits into an integrated performance conditioning programme. I often find myself looking at a rather perplexed face staring back at me when I send an athlete home from training to get some additional rest. I can tell from their faces that they think I'm mad. 'The fitness coach is telling me to have rest, there must be a catch, surely I should be training!' Knowing when to take time out from training to recover is really important and we will cover the optimal recovery strategies later on in the book. For now, just remember that Hans Selye says it's OK to take time out from training to recover.

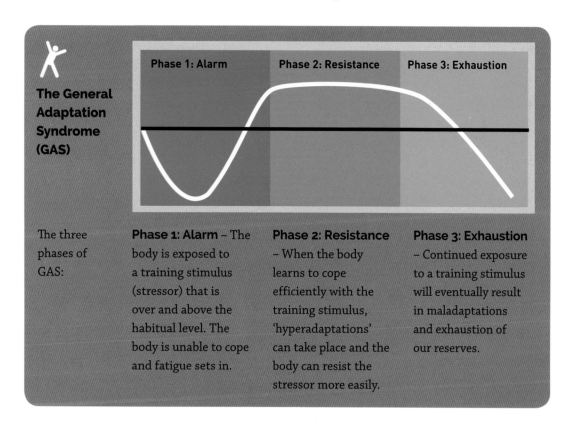

The General Adaptation Syndrome (GAS)

Phase 1: Alarm Phase 2: Resistance Phase 3: Exhaustion

The three phases of GAS:

Phase 1: Alarm – The body is exposed to a training stimulus (stressor) that is over and above the habitual level. The body is unable to cope and fatigue sets in.

Phase 2: Resistance – When the body learns to cope efficiently with the training stimulus, 'hyperadaptations' can take place and the body can resist the stressor more easily.

Phase 3: Exhaustion – Continued exposure to a training stimulus will eventually result in maladaptations and exhaustion of our reserves.

PROGRESSIVE OVERLOAD

❛A training adaptation only takes place if the magnitude of training load is above the habitual level.❜

Zatsiorsky & Kraemer, 2006

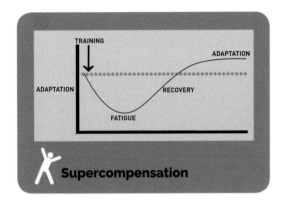

Supercompensation

This cornerstone of training links nicely to the accommodation cornerstone discussed earlier, but we need to go back to ancient Greece – to the 6th century BC, in fact – to find the mythical origins of this cornerstone. Milo was a wrestler; his strength and fitness levels were legendary and he won pretty much every tournament that he competed in. To become the greatest wrestler in Greece (he won six Olympic titles) he had to train. Legend has it that as a young child he would carry a newborn calf to and from the pasture every day. He did this day after day, week after week, and month after month. The calf became a fully grown ox over time, and as the calf grew the load Milo carried increased progressively (progressive overload).

We know we can't do the same thing over and over again and expect to see improvements in fitness and performance. Our body is pretty strange when you think about it, in that it actually needs a bit of stress on the system in order to adapt. When we complete a tough training session, the body says 'If he's going to do that to me again, I need to be ready', and it sets off a chain of events that will eventually result in a training adaptation, so that the next time it's confronted with a tough training session it's ready and waiting. Your training has to be designed to progressively overload the body systems and fuel stores and it must be applied carefully to improve performance. Progressive overload provides a stimulus to enhance physical, physiological and performance outcomes. Overload can be produced through the management of acute training variables (sets, reps, load, recovery etc) and we will cover this in more detail later in the book.

REVERSIBILITY

Use it or lose it, that's about as complicated as it gets! I've often found myself talking to someone who wants to get back in shape and they tell me that it shouldn't be too difficult because back in the day they used to play (insert any sport played at school) for their county. The problem is, that was 15 years ago and the prime athletic specimen that graced the county rugby pitch has long since departed and been replaced by a middle-aged man with a middle-age spread!

When we stop training, the fitness levels we have worked hard to develop will drop. There are differences between fitness qualities in terms of the level of de-training that occurs over time; some fall away quicker than others. How quickly fitness levels drop depends on several factors, including chronological age, previous fitness levels and training history, but the changes can occur pretty quickly.

Aerobic capacity can drop by as much as 20 per cent during a 3-week period and muscle mass can drop by up to 30 per cent after just a month.

If you have a significant training history you will maintain fitness levels longer than beginners, but they won't stick around for ever! Reversibility is an important consideration when coming back from prolonged periods of inactivity, either through choice (holiday) or enforced (injury). When you return to training you can't just start at your previous level, you need to build your training back up to previous standards over time.

SPECIFICITY

SAID (Specific Adaptation to Imposed Demands) is a training principle that links closely to functionality of training, which we discussed earlier in this section when looking at the five-point blueprint for success. In the past, coaches and athletes have run away with the idea of specificity and taken it to mean that training needs to look and feel like the sporting event itself. This is not the case and is a misinterpretation. If it were true then the only type of training athletes would need to do would be the sport itself and we know that just doesn't cut it any more.

Remember that a certain exercise or type of training produces adaptations specific to the activity performed and only in the muscles (and energy systems) that are stressed by the activity. When developing training programmes and selecting training methods, consider the degree of metabolic or mechanical symmetry between exercise type and performance outcome, as well as the degree to which a training exercise as part of a programme affects the long-term performance improvement (transfer of training effect). The basic mechanics, not the outward appearance of the training methods, are the most important factors when considering specificity and transfer. Squatting may not look like an exercise with a high degree of specificity for a golfer, but developing strength in the lower limbs will improve the golfer's functional capacity (improved strength, better balance, increased range of motion) and have a positive performance impact over the long term.

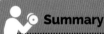 **Summary**

Developing a modern-day training programme must have a logical and systematic approach. An integrated performance conditioning (IPC) programme is a comprehensive system of preparation designed to deliver improved levels of functional capacity. A structured programme of physical preparation will provide a systematic progression in your training and allow you to realise your performance outcomes. Now you understand the fundamentals of integrated performance conditioning and the cornerstones of physical preparation that underpin programme design and training adaptations, we can move on and discover exactly how you can train like an athlete.

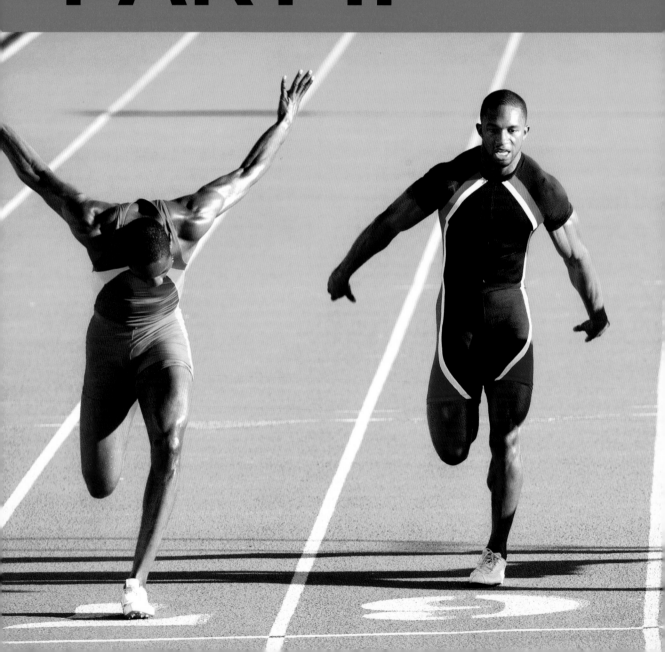

PART II

TRAINING LIKE AN ATHLETE

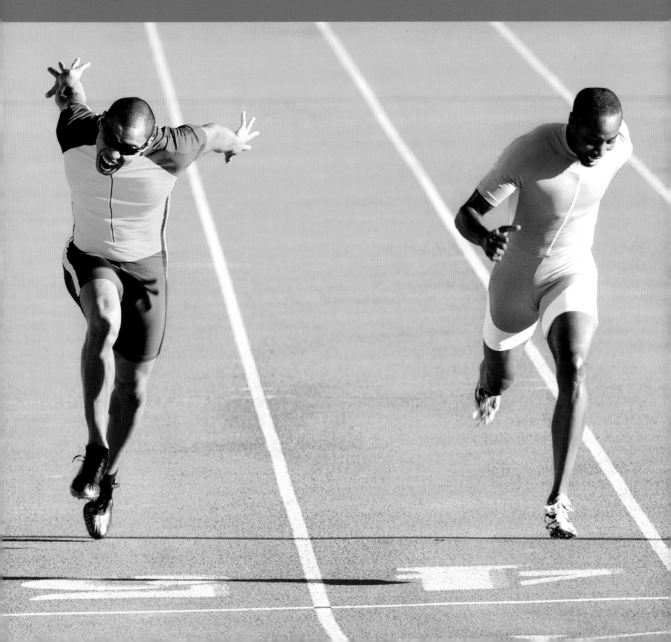

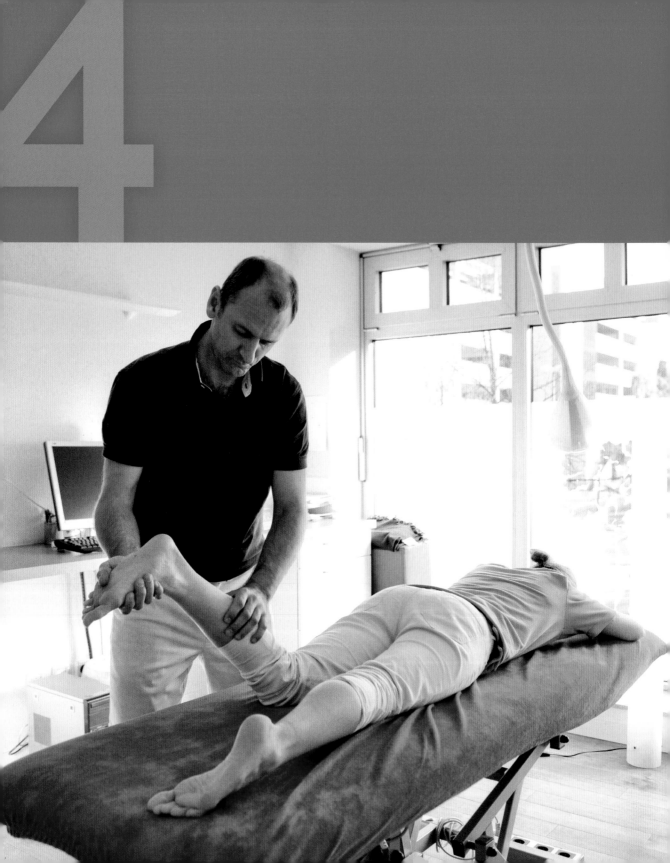

4

INJURY REDUCTION

Previous injury combined with inadequate or non-existent rehabilitation will set you up for further injury.

If I had one pound for every athlete I treated who only took injury prevention work seriously after suffering a serious injury I would have retired years ago!!!!

Grant Downie OBE, MCSP HCPC. Head of Performance, Manchester City FC Academy

Injuries present a huge challenge to professional and recreational athletes. They are one of the biggest hindrances to consistent progression and, in the case of the recreational athlete and fitness enthusiast, are often the factor that will force them to quit. If you've had an injury, you will know that it ruins motivation and can lead to significant performance decrements. If you are not healthy, you can't train to the best of your ability, and progress will be limited.

Following an injury, you will always be 'load compromised' (you will have to consider the training loads that you place on your body more carefully) and this will influence both short- and long-term training

recommendations. This is not a place where you want to be!

Bill Knowles, a highly respected injury rehabilitation specialist, views an injury as an opportunity to redevelop strengths and skills during a period where performance has been compromised, and he believes everyone has the chance to become better during the process of what he calls the 'comeback'. Rather than wait for you to become injured before we address your fundamental movements, I would like to get on the front foot and work on reducing your potential for picking up an injury in the first place.

Most injuries can be prevented if controlled early in the training programme. When your body is talking to you, listen. It will tell you long before it's too late. You're out running when you notice a slight twinge in your knee. Should you stop? Should you ignore it and push through? Catching a 'niggle' and addressing the problem will stop that niggle turning into an injury that eventually stops you training and competing. This doesn't mean you have to stop completely, but a slight twinge is probably your body saying, 'Hey, you need to be aware that I am starting to break down.'

Injuries occur because fundamentally the musculoskeletal system can't cope with the demands being placed upon it. Sure, if we look deep into the research we can find all sorts of interesting variables that could increase the risk of injury (hormone release, Q angles, gender) but these are often things we don't have any direct control over. What we can control is the condition of our musculoskeletal system by adopting a good programme of physical preparation.

Sports movements require jumping, sprinting, multiple changes of direction and rapid accelerations and decelerations. Overtraining, poor neuromuscular control, poor biomechanics and previous injuries all contribute to many of the injuries that stop

your training in its tracks. The good news is that many of your potential injury problems can be controlled or prevented, if you take action early.

I'm sure that many of you reading this book are capable of performing high-level activities, even though you possibly lack the appropriate level of gross athleticism and are inefficient in the fundamental movements. Adopt a long-term approach to physical preparation. Many of the clients I work with are highly skilled in their sport but often lack the physical competencies required to withstand its demands. The key message – start conditioning early!

Many of you will also choose to train around a pre-existing problem or simply do not train your weaknesses. In the short term this may not seem to be a problem, but if you layer year after year of poor movement patterns while training around a pre-existing problem and simply not training your weaknesses, you'll end up with a chronic overuse injury and potentially an acute injury that stops you in your tracks.

The focus of this section is on injury reduction rather than rehabilitation. This is a subtle but important distinction to make. This section is not a replacement for a good sports physiotherapist! Rehabilitation following an injury requires a very particular skill set and if you've already picked up an injury you should find a good physiotherapist to work with as soon as possible. Not unlike the main character played by Liam Neeson in the film *Taken*, physiotherapists *'have a very particular set of*

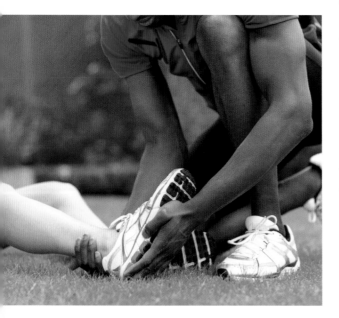

◁ Injury is an opportunity

SHIN PAIN

Shin pain is a common problem and can be caused by one or more components. If your shin pain is due to inflammation, you will typically experience pain along the inside border of the tibia (shin). The discomfort usually decreases with warming up, but comes back after rest. If your pain increases with exercise and is accompanied by a tight feeling, but disappears quickly post exercise, then the problem may be compartment syndrome. If your pain comes on gradually and is aggravated by exercise, you could have a bone strain (stress reaction). Often, the pain increases when jumping or you'll experience localised tenderness over the tibia (shin). You may also experience pain at rest or a 'night ache'.

Common Causes

- Increase in activity (training volume, mileage, speed, gradient)
- Decrease in recovery time between training sessions
- Changes of surface
- Change of footwear (lower heel, high heel tab)
- Lack of conditioning (poor lower limb strength)
- Movement dysfunction (poor running mechanics)

▽ Many running based injuries can be linked to sudden changes in training volumes

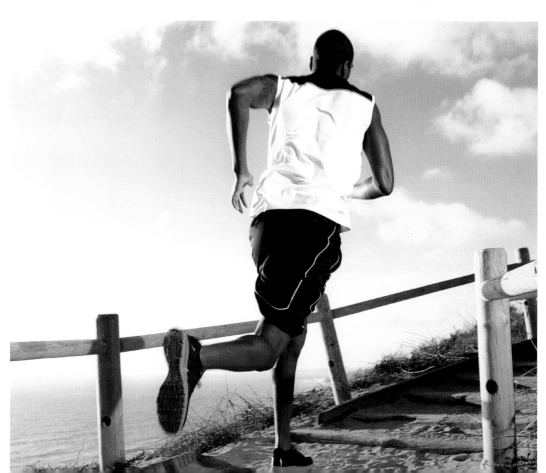

INJURY REDUCTION STRATEGIES – LOWER LEG, ANKLE AND FOOT

Problems at the lower leg, ankle and foot have a habit of showing up elsewhere in the body (typically the knees and hips), so it makes sense to spend time working on some simple injury reduction strategies that you can incorporate into your training programme to reduce the likelihood of them occurring and derailing your training.

INJURY REDUCTION - LOWER LEG ANKLE AND FOOT - 1				
Order	**Exercise**		**Sets**	**Reps**	**Coaching Cue**
1	Myofascial release	Plantar Fascia	-	-	spend 1-2 minutes per self-myofascial release technique
		Calf	-	-	
		Tibialis Anterior	-	-	
2	Eccentric Knee Squat		1 - 3	3 - 5 ea	front, left, right represents 1 rep
3	Dynamic Achilles Stretch		1 - 3	3 - 5 ea	feel a stretch on your right calf achillies
4	Calf Raise	Gastrocnemius	2 - 3	10 - 15	push evenly through the entire width of your foot
		Soleus	2 - 3	10 - 15	
5	Ankle Jumps	In place	2 - 4	10	fully extend the ankles on each jump
6	SL Balance		2 - 3	30 - 60s ea	maintain your balance with minimal movement

INJURY REDUCTION - LOWER LEG ANKLE AND FOOT - 2				
Order	**Exercise**		**Sets**	**Reps**	**Coaching Cue**
1	Myofascial release	Plantar Fascia	-	-	spend 1-2 minutes per self-myofascial release technique
		Calf	-	-	
		Tibialis Anterior	-	-	
2	3D - Stretch	Gastrocnemius	1 - 3	30 - 60s	change the orientation of limbs every 10-30 seconds
3		Soleus	1 - 3	30 - 60s	
4	Calf Raise	Eccentrics	2 - 3	10 - 15	push evenly through the entire width of your foot
		Drops	2 - 3	10	
5	Ankle Jumps	Forward	2 - 4	10	fully extend the ankles on each jump
6	Eccentric Reach		1 - 3	3 - 5 ea	maintain your balance with minimal movement

INJURY REDUCTION - LOWER LEG ANKLE AND FOOT - 3				
Order	**Exercise**		**Sets**	**Reps**	**Coaching Cue**
1	Myofascial release	Plantar Fascia	-	-	spend 1-2 minutes per self-myofascial release technique
		Calf	-	-	
		Tibialis Anterior	-	-	
2	3D - Stretch	Gastrocnemius	1 - 3	30 - 60s	change the orientation of the limbs every 10-30 seconds
		Soleus	1 - 3	30 - 60s	
3	Calf Raise	Gastrocnemius	2 - 3	10 - 15	push evenly through the entire width of your foot
		Drops	2 - 3	10 - 15	
4	Ankle Jumps	Lateral	2 - 4	10	fully extend
5	SL Balance and Reach	Forward	1 - 3	3 - 5ea	maintain your balance with minimal movement

Lower leg, ankle and foot injury reduction sessions

Knee

Running-based activities cause a lot of problems relating to the lower limb, with the knee proving to be one of the areas most susceptible to injury. So if your sport of choice involves running, jumping and changing direction in some form or other, you need to pay special attention to your knees and the surrounding structures. While some of the knee injuries we discuss in this section are sometimes unavoidable, you can reduce your risk of an injury by avoiding sudden increases in training frequency, duration, or intensity of exercise and incorporating the injury reduction programme outlined at the end of this section into your weekly training schedule.

 Common Problems

- Patellofemoral Pain Syndrome (PFPS)
- Anterior Cruciate Ligament (ACL) Injuries
- Meniscal Tears
- Medial Collateral Ligament (MCL) Injuries

PATELLOFEMORAL PAIN SYNDROME (PFPS)

PFPS is one of the most common diagnoses and this is probably due to the fact that it's somewhat of an all-encompassing term for pain around the kneecap (anterior knee pain). PFPS is a common and sometimes debilitating problem that can be difficult to treat. Pain in the knee region is provoked when the kneecap fails to track properly in a groove on the thigh bone called the patellofemoral groove. Poor 'tracking' of the kneecap results in abnormal stresses on the under-surface of the patella, which can cause anterior knee pain. You'll experience pain at the front of the knee and just sitting for extended periods of time can bring on symptoms. Walking down stairs and running will also be painful.

Common Causes

- Tight hip, calf, hamstring and iliotibial band
- Lack of strength in supporting structures (muscles) surrounding the knee and hip and an imbalance between the muscles that form the quadriceps (four muscles that extend the knee and support the patella)
- Movement dysfunction (static or dynamic lower limb malalignment, altered hip, knee or foot posture)
- Anatomic variations, such as a shallow patellofemoral groove or increased Q angle

ANTERIOR CRUCIATE LIGAMENT (ACL) INJURIES

The ACL plays a key role in the stabilisation of the knee and is particularly susceptible to injury during rapid deceleration and changes of direction. Three movements that can often result in an ACL injury are:

- Change of direction
- Landing with a straight knee
- Landing on one leg and hyperextending the knee

An ACL injury can strike both men and women but research shows that women competing in sport are more vulnerable (four to six times) than their male counterparts. An ACL injury can take anything between 6 and 36 months to come back from, so it's definitely one to try to avoid!

Common Causes

- Movement dysfunction (knee valgus or 'kissing knees', poor landing mechanics, 'heavy' or 'stiff' landings)
- Lack of strength in supporting structures (muscles) surrounding the knee and hip, including the hamstrings (who would have thought that the muscles at the back of the leg could help reduce the chances of a knee injury!)
- Anatomic variations, especially for females whose pelvic anatomy (wider hips) results in an increased Q angle

MENISCAL TEARS

The knee joint contains a medial meniscus (on the inside of the knee joint) and lateral meniscus (on the outside of the knee joint). The meniscal cartilages are essentially squidgy cushions of cartilage that act like shock absorbers and contribute to the smooth movement and stability of the knee. If you're going to tear a meniscus, the chances are it will be the medial mensiscus (five times more likely) and meniscal tears often go hand in hand with an ACL tear.

Common Causes

- Twisting or pivoting while the foot is anchored to the ground (think rugby, football, basketball and skiing)
- Receiving a blow to the outside of the knee, forcing it inwards
- Movement dysfunction (poor landing mechanics, 'heavy' or 'stiff' landings) or poor deceleration qualities

MEDIAL COLLATERAL LIGAMENT (MCL) INJURIES

The MCL extends from the end of the thigh bone to the top of the shin bone on the inside of the knee. If you're aged 20–34 and enjoy playing contact sports or have to perform quick changes in direction (skiers, hockey, football, basketball and tennis players), you'll have an increased chance of picking up an MCL injury. MCL injuries are unavoidable, but you can reduce your risk by avoiding sudden increases in training frequency, duration, or intensity of exercise.

Common Causes

- Contact sports in which an opponent falls on the outside of the knee joint
- Sudden force or twisting to the outside of the knee during rapid changes of direction
- Movement dysfunction (poor landing strategies and poor deceleration qualities)
- Lack of strength in supporting structures (muscles) surrounding the knee

INJURY REDUCTION STRATEGIES – KNEE

Let's face it, some knee injuries are unavoidable, but you can reduce your risk of picking up a nasty one by working on your single-leg strength. Single-leg strength is possibly one of the most important qualities in injury reduction strategies for knee injuries. We spend a significant amount of time on one leg (approximately 55 per cent during walking and up to 85 per cent when running), so it makes intuitive sense for you to spend some of your time when training developing single-leg strength.

INJURY REDUCTION - KNEE - 1					
Order	Exercise		Sets	Reps	Coaching Cue
1	Myofascial release and 3D - Stretch	Gluteals	-	-	spend 1-2 minutes per self-myofascial release and 3D - stretch technique
		Hamstrings	-	-	
		Quadriceps/Hip Flexors	-	-	
		Iliotibial Band (ITB)	-	-	
		Tensor Fascia Latae (TFL)	-	-	
2	Mini-Band	Athletic	1 - 2	10 ea	controlled movement
		Tall	1 - 2	10 ea	
		Lying Hip Abduction	3 - 4	5	
3	4-Point Hip Extension		3 - 4	5 ea	avoid movement through the lower back
4	Bridge		2 - 4	8 - 12	squeeze gluteals at top like two fists
5	Single Leg Squat		3 - 4	5 - 8 ea	maintain knee alignment

INJURY REDUCTION - KNEE - 2					
Order	Exercise		Sets	Reps	Coaching Cue
1	Myofascial release and 3D - Stretch	Gluteals	-	-	spend 1-2 minutes per self-myofascial release and 3D - stretch technique
		Hamstrings	-	-	
		Quadriceps/Hip Flexors	-	-	
		Iliotibial Band (ITB)	-	-	
		Tensor Fascia Latae (TFL)	-	-	
2	Mini-Band	Offset	1 - 2	10 ea	controlled movement
		Diagonal	1 - 2	10 ea	
		Lying Hip Abduction	3 - 4	5	
3	4-Point Hip Extension		3 - 4	5 ea	avoid movement through the lower back
4	3-Point Bridge		2 - 4	8 - 12 ea	squeeze gluteals at top like two fists
5	Single Leg Squat		3 - 4	5 - 8	maintain knee alignment

INJURY REDUCTION - KNEE - 3					
Order	Exercise		Sets	Reps	Coaching Cue
1	Myofascial release and 3D - Stretch	Gluteals	-	-	spend 1-2 minutes per self-myofascial release and 3D - stretch technique
		Hamstrings	-	-	
		Quadriceps/Hip Flexors	-	-	
		Iliotibial Band (ITB)	-	-	
		Tensor Fascia Latae (TFL)	-	-	
2	Mini-Band	Box	1 - 2	10 ea	controlled movement
		Step and Squat	1 - 2	10 ea	
		Hip Activation	3 - 4	5	
3	4-Point Hip Extension		3 - 4	5 ea	avoid movement through the lower back
4	Bridge		2 - 4	8 - 12	squeeze gluteals at top like two fists
5	Single Leg Squat		3 - 4	5 - 8	maintain knee alignment

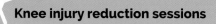 **Knee injury reduction sessions**

Regardless of training levels, men are naturally stronger, so women need to embrace strength training and get stronger, rather than avoid it.

Ensure your injury reduction programme includes rotational multidimensional training exercises and include elements of CHAOS in your training. Robert dos Remedios has coined the term 'CHAOS training' to reflect the open skills that he uses to develop speed, strength and control in his athletes (in 10 years he has coached thousands of collegiate athletes and has only had three ACL injuries – one male, two female – that's a pretty impressive record if you ask me!).

Shoulder

Shoulder injuries are common and can be persistent in nature, eventually leading to degenerative changes and chronic injury problems. Repetitive overhead activities (throwing, catching, swimming) can overload the shoulder muscles, leading to pain and dysfunction. Poor posture (rounded shoulders and forward head position) can compound issues.

COMMON PROBLEMS: ROTATOR CUFF INJURIES

The rotator cuff is a group of four muscles (supraspinatus, infraspinatus, subscapularis, teres minor) that extend from your scapula (shoulder blade) to the head of the humerus (top of your upper arm) and they work as a team to provide movement and stability to the shoulder joint.

Common Causes

- Overuse due to repetitive or unaccustomed overhead activities such as throwing, catching, swimming (freestyle and butterfly), painting or heavy lifting and other activities involving repetitive movements of the shoulder
- Instability and poor control of the scapula (shoulder blade)
- Muscle imbalances and lack of appropriate conditioning of the rotator cuff muscles resulting in early onset of fatigue and movement dysfunction

Common rotator cuff injuries include:

- Rotator cuff tendonitis – acute onset of pain due to irritation and inflammation of the tendon
- Impingement syndrome – irritation and inflammation of the tendon(s), leading to chronic pain in the shoulder
- Swimmer's shoulder – caused by repetitive overhead movements combined with movement dysfunction due to muscle imbalances
- Rugby shoulder – caused by intense tackling
- Thrower's shoulder – caused by repetitive movements compounded by movement dysfunction due to muscle imbalances

INJURY REDUCTION STRATEGIES – SHOULDER

One thing you're not going to find as part of your injury reduction strategy for the shoulder is a bunch of exercises that attempt to isolate specific muscles around the shoulder. Renowned strength and conditioning coach Mike Boyle hits the nail on the head: 'Most upper body injuries are linked to a lack of balance.' What does he mean? Mike is telling you quite clearly that the majority of the problems we've discussed in the section relating to the rotator cuff can be traced back to an imbalance and lack of conditioning between the muscles at the front of the body (the ones you see in the mirror) and the ones at the back of the body (the ones you never look at and therefore don't bother to train). The shoulder is a complex joint, but rather than get caught up in minutiae, keep it simple and develop well-conditioned shoulders and back using some simple exercises outlined below.

INJURY REDUCTION - SHOULDER - 1					
Order	**Exercise**		**Sets**	**Reps**	**Coaching Cue**
1	Myofascial release	Thoracic	-	-	spend 1-2 minutes on thoracic release
2	3D - Stretch	Back	1 - 3	30 - 60s	change the orientation of the limbs every 10-30 seconds
		Chest	1 - 3	30 - 60s	
3	Shoulder Circle		2 - 3	5 - 10 ea	large circles, full range of motion
4	PNF Diagonal		2 - 3	5 - 10 ea	large movements, full range of motion
5	Figure 8		2 - 3	5 - 10 ea	large controlled movements

INJURY REDUCTION - SHOULDER - 2					
Order	**Exercise**		**Sets**	**Reps**	**Coaching Cue**
1	Myofascial release	Thoracic	-	-	spend 1-2 minutes on thoracic release
2	3D - Stretch	Back	1 - 3	30 - 60s	change the orientation of the limbs every 10-30 seconds
		Chest	1 - 3	30 - 60s	
3	RTW's		1 - 2	10 ea	large, controlled movement
4	Flutters		2 - 3	5 ea	initiate movement from shoulder blades
5	YTWL		1 - 2	5 - 8 ea	controlled movements

INJURY REDUCTION - SHOULDER - 3					
Order	**Exercise**		**Sets**	**Reps**	**Coaching Cue**
1	Myofascial release	Thoracic	-	-	spend 1-2 minutes on thoracic release
2	3D - Stretch	Back	1 - 3	30 - 60s	change the orientation of the limbs every 10-30 seconds
		Chest	1 - 3	30 - 60s	
3	Truck Drivers		1 - 2	5 - 8 ea	controlled movement
4	Shoulder Shuffles		1 - 2	30 - 60s	keep tension on the mini-band
5	X-Band Walks		2 - 3	10 ea	focus on maintaining posture

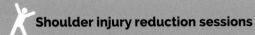 **Shoulder injury reduction sessions**

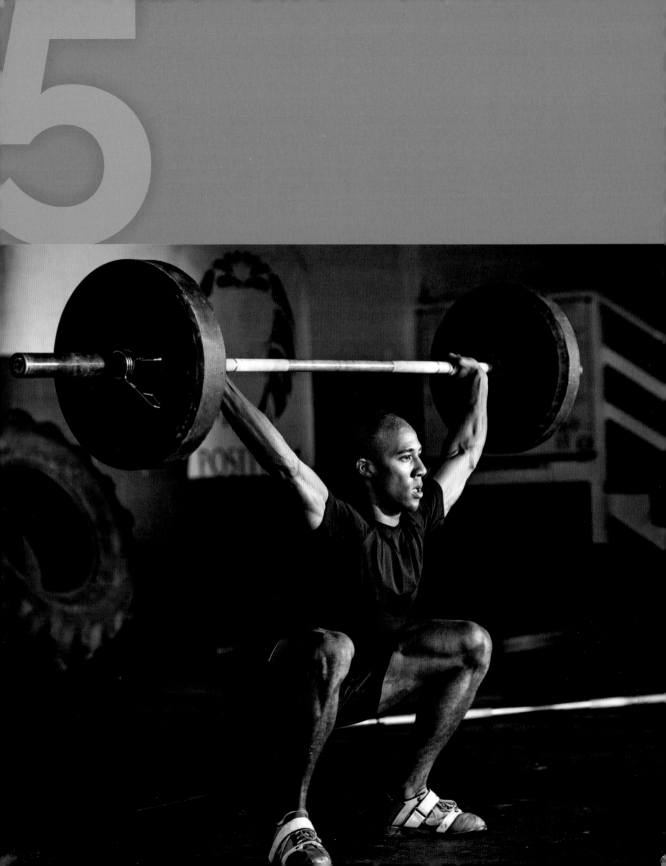

MOVEMENT QUALITY TRAINING

■ **We know from the first section of the book,** in which we explored the importance of developing gross athleticism, that the most successful athletes are the ones with the largest movement vocabulary.

If we have good fundamental movement patterns (letters of the alphabet), we can link them together to produce more complex and challenging movements (words) and develop an extensive 'movement vocabulary' that we can use in day-to-day and sporting activities. Developing the 'functional capacity' needed to improve and deliver performance is vital

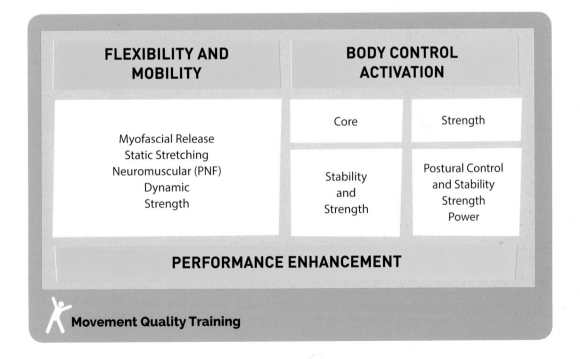

FLEXIBILITY AND MOBILITY

BODY CONTROL ACTIVATION

Myofascial Release
Static Stretching
Neuromuscular (PNF)
Dynamic
Strength

Core

Strength

Stability
and
Strength

Postural Control
and Stability
Strength
Power

PERFORMANCE ENHANCEMENT

Movement Quality Training

for success and MQT is an excellent way of preparing the body so you can maximise the active ranges of motion required for fluid, athletic movement.

'There is one common denominator in all sport and that is "Movement". My strategy for coaching quality movement is quite simple. Help the athlete to "discover and feel" their optimal biomechanical positions, and then ask them to reproduce the "feeling" again and again. After all, you cannot reproduce something unless you have first experienced it.'

Mark Spivey B.App.Sci. (Human Movement/Sports Science) ASCC. Director of Fitness and Sport, Radley College (United Kingdom)

We all share common movement patterns that need to be developed: squat, hinge, pull (vertical and horizontal), push (vertical and horizontal), lunge, carry, reach, lift, accelerate and decelerate. Movement is something that should develop and improve as we get older, but many clients and athletes find themselves trying to perform complex movements with a limited movement vocabulary through a combination of factors such as lifestyle, work, sedentary living, injury and illness. Compound movement dysfunction with poor or non-existent physical preparation programmes and you are leaving a lot of your untapped potential on the gym floor.

> Your body is a highly complex organism and if you want to be capable of delivering fluid, athletic movements, you need to work on developing gross athleticism.

Movement Quality Training

- Reinforces correct motor patterns
- Proprioception and body control
- Synchronisation to finely coordinate movement and motor function
- Increased kinaesthetic awareness
- Technical reinforcement
- Skill rehearsal

Including MQT sessions in your day-to-day training will reinforce the correct postures and positions of the body in order to allow for effective transfer and expression of force and power. Performing MQT activities can improve proprioception (the ability to sense changes from within the body regarding position, motion and equilibrium) and body control by causing increased sensitivity in the body's mechanoreceptors (sensors that respond to pressure, vibration, stretching and other mechanical stimuli). These receptors work together to finely coordinate movement and motor function relative to the external environment that the body is experiencing. Activation of these receptors is crucial for exercise and sport, as a greater awareness of the position of one's own body allows for increased kinaesthetic awareness, giving you more control over your movement. MQT also allows for skill rehearsal, which reinforces the correct motor patterns that will be carried out when participating in the ensuing exercise activity.You'll also develop core stability and strength, while at the same time improving balance and coordination in all planes of motion.

In addition to kinaesthetic regulation of movement, the psychological side of MQT is also important elsewhere. Stimulating the mind through more complex movement tasks often allows for 'technical reinforcement' of an activity and/or movement patterns that will be experienced in an ensuing activity. Technical reinforcement is an added bonus of MQT.

'Establish functional mobility first, as quality proprioception is not possible with limited mobility!'

Duncan French PhD, ASCC, CSCS, ASCA-L2. Technical Lead for Strength & Conditioning, English Institute of Sport

Movement Quality Pathway

MQT encompasses a range of training interventions using a four-step process of release, activation, integration and reinforcement. A comprehensive MQT session will address all elements, but the exact proportion will depend on your individual needs. If you have poor core stability, you will need to develop this aspect of your fitness before focusing too much time and energy on higher-level activities. MQT is an excellent way of preparing the body in a way that maximises the active ranges of motion required for fluid, athletic movement. It is a

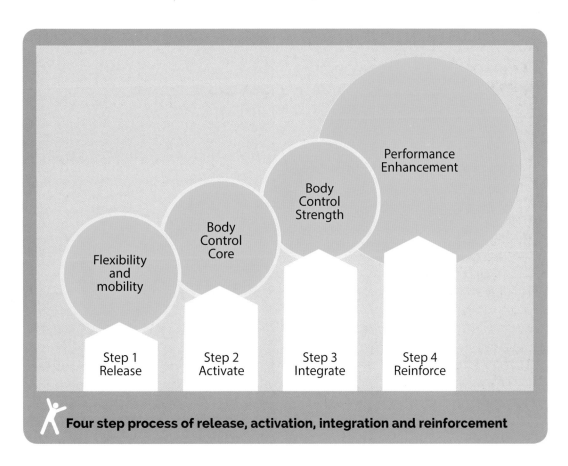

Flexibility and mobility

Body Control Core

Body Control Strength

Performance Enhancement

Step 1 Release

Step 2 Activate

Step 3 Integrate

Step 4 Reinforce

Four step process of release, activation, integration and reinforcement

concept that reiterates the correct postures and positions of the body in order to allow for effective transfer and expression of force and power.

Optimising movement for sports performance simply comes down to the ability to produce the right movement, at the right time, in the most efficient fashion possible … at speed!

Duncan French PhD, ASCC, CSCS, ASCA-L2. Technical Lead for Strength & Conditioning, English Institute of Sport

Step One – Release

Stretching is an exercise aimed at changing the structural extensibility of the muscle complex (muscle and associated connective tissue).

Castella, 1996

Flexibility training is directed towards increasing joint ROM, which may or may not include stretching exercises, but also includes exercises that alter the nervous system control of the muscles to allow greater motion to take place in the joints.

Bill Hartman

Mobility is the combination of muscle flexibility, joint range of motion and a body segment's freedom of movement.

Gray Cook

FLEXIBILITY AND MOBILITY

Flexibility and mobility training is often forgotten, misunderstood and misapplied. Poor levels of functional flexibility (I don't expect you all to be able to do the splits, we are looking for 'optimal' not 'maximal' range of motion!) can have a negative impact on your movement capacity and reduce your ability to move efficiently and effectively. However, an appropriate level of flexibility and mobility has the ability to allow you to move smoothly and easily through unrestricted, pain-free functional movements commonly seen in day-to-day and sporting situations. When incorporating flexibility and mobility into an MQT programme, you are primarily concerned with developing acute (elastic) adaptations.

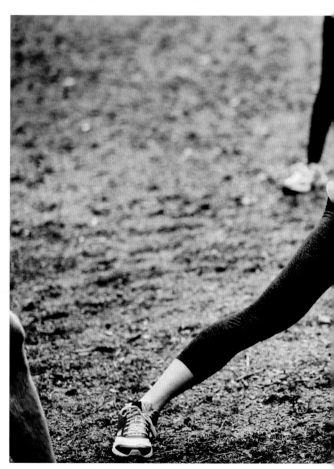

This type of adaptation is really getting your body primed for the next activity (training session) and ensuring you are ready to hit all the correct postures and positions and have the appropriate level of functional flexibility and mobility to make the right 'shapes'. If you need to develop range of motion, you will need to have a specific 'developmental' session built in as part of your long-term training programme. The best way to improve your functional flexibility and mobility is to adopt a multi-modal approach, and there are several options available to you.

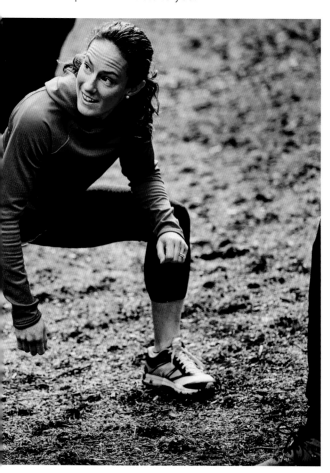

'*A hallmark of elite sports performance is efficient athletic movement, whichever your chosen sport at the highest level the best athletes just seem to make it look so easy!*'

Steve Wright Chartered Physiotherapist, Certified Kinetic Control Movement Therapist. Senior Physiotherapist, English Premier League

SOFT TISSUE WORK

Self-Myofascial Release (SMR) is a relatively simple technique that you can use to alleviate trigger points. With simple and inexpensive pieces of equipment (foam roller, massage stick, tennis or hockey ball) you will be able to maintain tissue quality, allowing you to train more effectively without breaking down. You will find a simple SMR routine in the exercise reference section of the book.

STRETCHING
Static

Static stretching is one of the safest forms of flexibility training, resulting in less muscle soreness and providing more relief from muscular distress. This type of stretching is great for improving range of motion but shouldn't typically be used as part of your movement preparation or cool-down routine. Static stretching can be:

1. Gravity assisted (no muscle contraction)
2. Partner assisted (no muscle contraction)
3. Load assisted (no muscle contraction)

You will find a simple series of static stretches in the exercise reference section of the book.

◁ Poor levels of functional flexibility can have a negative impact on your movement capacity

Dynamic

Dynamic stretching is a more active movement typically incorporated into the warm-up and cool-down, moving the muscle through a range of motion into some tension and then back out again. This form of flexibility training is great for getting the body ready for action but if this is the only sort of flexibility training you use, you will not improve flexibility. It is a good way of taking your body through active range of motion and can be used as part of your movement preparation or cool-down routine. Dynamic stretching can include:

- Functional movements
- Hurdle work (sway under, forward and backward walkover)
- Squat and lunge patterns
- Movement complexes

You will find a series of simple dynamic stretches in the exercise reference section of the book.

Proprioceptive Neuromuscular Facilitation (PNF)

PNF stretching can be very effective and uses muscle contractions prior to a stretch in order to bring about maximum relaxation. There are nine different methods of PNF stretching, but my personal favourite is the Hold-Relax (HR) technique, for which you contract your muscles against a static resistance (usually a partner helping you with the stretch) from a point at which you are experiencing limitations in your range of motion. You hold that contraction for a brief period (5–15 seconds) before relaxing, during which time your partner moves your limb into a newly gained range of motion.

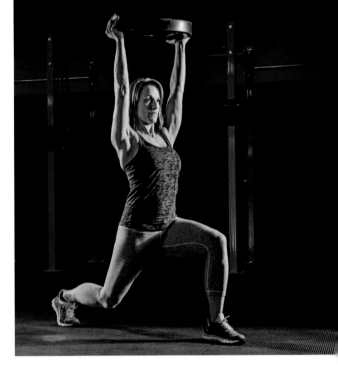

△ Strength training can improve functional flexibility

STRENGTH

Active range of motion will not always change with static stretching due to a lack of strength at a specific point in the range of motion. Use of functional movements that you complete in day-to-day life (squat or lunge patterns, etc) is an effective strategy to develop flexibility and will improve soft tissue extensibility and enhance neuromuscular control through a full range of multidimensional movement. You will find a series of simple strength training exercises that can be used to improve range of motion in the exercise reference section of the book.

'If an athlete is not strong "enough" for their bodyweight and stature, it is impossible for them to become agile.'

Duncan French PhD, ASCC, CSCS, ASCA-L2. Technical Lead for Strength & Conditioning, English Institute of Sport

Step Two – Activate

The term 'core' is widely misunderstood. An integrated MQT programme should develop appropriate levels of core stability and strength so you can produce multidimensional actions quickly and efficiently during functional movements. This can be achieved by developing appropriate levels of conditioning across all three areas: local stabilisation, global stabilisation and functional movement.

'Think about the outcome of the movement rather than the muscles being used – train the movement, not the muscle. Remember, new range is weak range – be strong throughout.'

Darren Roberts High Performance Manager, Harris and Ross Healthcare

LOCAL STABILISATION

The deeper, smaller muscles, such as the transversus abdominis, internal oblique, lumbar multifidus, pelvic floor muscles and diaphragm, play a vital role in creating spinal stability. These provide 'segmental stability', preventing excessive compressive, shear and rotational forces in the spine. These muscles have important functional roles during sitting, standing, lying and walking, but they cannot provide spinal stability during rapid actions.

 Typical Exercises

Isometric holds (planks, side holds, bridges), foot slides, dead bugs, supermans, bird dogs, plank marches.

GLOBAL STABILISATION

Larger muscles, including the quadratus lumborum, psoas major, external oblique, rectus abdominis, gluteus medius and adductors, attach to the pelvis and spine and work together to produce movement. These muscles play an essential role in the transfer of force between the upper and lower body as well as stability between the pelvis and spine (flexion/extension, rotation, throwing/catching). While the ability to generate movement is important, an often overlooked quality is the ability to resist rather than create rotation, and you should also be able to prevent rotation and excessive movement.

'The ability to position your centre of mass, and then stabilise appropriately, often at speed or against resistance, can be a huge determinant in the quality and efficiency of athletic movement, and ultimately performance.'

Steve Wright Chartered Physiotherapist, Certified Kinetic Control Movement Therapist, Senior Physiotherapist, English Premier League

 Typical Exercises

Sit-ups, roll outs, band rotations, back extensions, barbell rotations, cable rotations, cable lifts, cable chops, vertical isometric holds, aleknas.

FUNCTIONAL MOVEMENT

Larger superficial muscles, such as the latissimus dorsi, hamstrings and quadriceps, produce force and absorb force and provide dynamic stability during multidimensional functional activity (flexion/extension, rotation, throwing/catching). These muscles play a vital role in supporting postures during complex multidimensional movements that continually change as a function of real-world and sporting situations.

 Typical Exercises

Medicine ball slams, overhead medicine ball throws, lateral medicine ball throws, barbell twists, Turkish get-ups, plate rotations, Russian twists, windmill

Step Three – Integrate
POSTURAL CONTROL AND STABILITY

Postural control is a dynamic quality and the development of gross athleticism, general conditioning and higher levels of strength will allow you to control posture while moving and expand the 'balance threshold', a term coined by renowned strength and conditioning coach Vern Gambetta to describe the distance moved outside of the base support without losing control of the centre of gravity. Developing this aspect of MQT will enhance your ability to:

■ Manipulate your centre of gravity and base of support
■ Develop fundamental physical movement competencies (force transfer, flexibility, mobility, strength and muscular endurance)

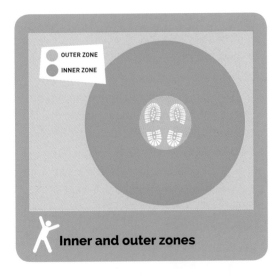

OUTER ZONE
INNER ZONE

Inner and outer zones

Exercise Progressions

■ **Inner Zone** (static, little joint movement, all body parts inside the base of support).
■ **Outer Zone** (dynamic, eccentric and concentric movements through larger ranges of motion, movement of body parts outside the base of support).

■ Develop and maintain appropriate joint control
■ Improve 'motor control'
■ Decrease stress on larger prime mover muscles while increasing stress on the smaller supporting muscles which are known as synergists.

Within each zone, exercises can be progressed by challenging stability:

■ Reduce the base of support, progressing from bilateral stance (two-leg) to unilateral stance (single-leg)

- Don't allow the arms or legs to act as a counterbalance
- Move the arms or legs in order to create movement and present a more dynamic stabilisation stimulus
- Close eyes or move head
- Change surfaces (stability cushions, balance beams etc)

 Typical Exercises

Single-leg balance, single-leg balance and reach (forward, lateral, back, unstable single-leg balance, unstable single-leg balance and reach)

STRENGTH

Strength training is an important part of the MQT process and exercises can be selected from across the functional continuum as described earlier in the book to develop fundamental movement skills that focus on quality of movement before quantity.

POWER

The ability to develop maximal force as quickly as possible enhances performance during athletic movements, and if you want to be able to move with precision, you must be able to load, stabilise and accelerate your musculoskeletal system. MQT training should incorporate exercises that require higher levels of eccentric strength, control and stability along with planned incorporation of acceleration and deceleration. Strength training involves:

- Detection and reaction to stimulus
- Dynamic movements
- Acceleration and deceleration
- Tumbling, dodging, hops and jumps

Step Four – Reinforce

In the final step of the movement quality pathway, performance enhancement activities involving application of the fundamentals of integrated performance conditioning should be used. At this stage it's all about incorporating multidimensional athletic movements designed to transfer into improved performance. Complex movement tasks should be used to develop 'technical reinforcement' of an activity and/or movement pattern that will be experienced in an ensuing activity.

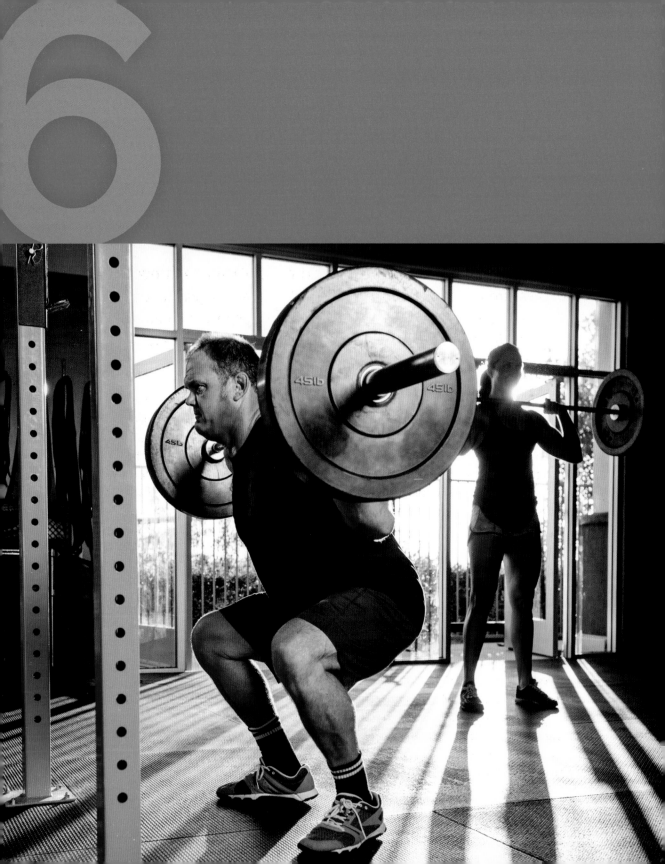

STRENGTH AND POWER

■ **For most fitness enthusiasts and recreational athletes,** the benefits of strength training are outweighed by a fear of gaining too much bulk, loss of flexibility and diminished 'feel' for their sport. Unfortunately, this thinking will stop you from reaping the benefits that a properly designed strength programme has to offer.

A well-designed strength programme will unlock your athletic potential. In this section, we will look at the best techniques for improving strength and power without compromising other aspects of training. But first let's answer the question, what exactly is strength?

> **Strength is the ability to generate or control force.**

Knowing the difference between strength and power training not only will give you a competitive performance advantage but undertaken correctly will for sure reduce injury rates … So maximise your performance gains!!

Grant Downie OBE, MCSP HCPC. Head of Performance, Manchester City FC Academy

We can actually produce and control force in a number of ways and in this section we will explore the different types of strength and how your approach to training will be dictated by the type of strength you want to develop. The human body has over 660 muscles (40–45 per cent of its total mass), which when combined with other connective tissues transmit force to the skeletal system to produce movement (Cardinale, Newton & Nosaka, 2011). When you follow a strength training programme, you will experience improvements due to: 1) neuromuscular adaptations (basically upgrading your body's internal internet from a dial-up service to fibre optic broadband); 2) increased cross-sectional area (CSA) (adding some extra meat on the bone, having a 10oz steak for dinner instead of a 6oz one); or 3) a combination of both.

"Keep your training simple! ... focus on "force production", "force reduction", and "stabilisation". That's strength training covered!"

Duncan French PhD, ASCC, CSCS, ASCA-L2. Technical Lead for Strength & Conditioning, English Institute of Sport

Strength and power training causes adaptive changes to various systems within the body, including the musculoskeletal system (structure of skeletal muscle, tendons), the neuromuscular system (contractile rate), neuroendocrine system (regulation of protein synthesis and muscle growth).

Benefits of Strength and Power Development

....

- Increased strength and power
- Improved neural functioning
- Increased rate of force development (RFD)
- Improved fine motor control
- Structural modifications in bone
- Improved tendon CSA and morphology
- Adaptive responses in testosterone, cortisol and growth hormone

Strength and power training ultimately leads to improved mechanical muscle function, which in turn results in improved functional performance in various activities of day-to-day life, including:

- Athletic performance
- General health

- Rehabilitation and reconditioning
- Counteraction of aging-induced muscle loss

"Understanding how to apply the correct training modality, the correct volume and intensity and correct timing of each intervention is the 'holy grail' of strength and power development."

Cardinale, Newton & Nosaka, 2011

As we begin to explore the concepts of strength and power development, keep in mind the cornerstones of training discussed in the integrated performance conditioning section:

- **Quality** – Develop fundamental movement skills that focus on quality of movement before quantity.
- **Functional** – The level of functionality is related to the performance outcome you want to achieve.
- **Efficient** – Training like an athlete means having a programme that uses the minimum 'dose' but delivers the maximum 'effect'.
- **Continuity** – Planned variations are essential to elicit adaptations – develop programmes with both short- and long-term aims in mind.
- **Recovery** – Recovery and regeneration is a fundamental component of an integrated performance training programme.

For a comprehensive overview of the cornerstones of training, refer to the integrated performance conditioning section.

What type of strength do you need?

Developing an appropriate strength training programme is based on three elements:

1. Understanding your strength requirements – does your sport require maximum strength or reactive strength?
2. Knowledge of the most appropriate training techniques in order to develop those strength requirements.
3. Understanding how these training strategies should be incorporated into a long-term plan (phase potentiation) – sequencing your training so that the performance gains in one training phase can enhance training and performance gains in the next training phase.

So you need to figure out what type of strength you need to work on, the best training technique, and how your training will produce results over the long term.

CONDITIONING

Conditioning refers to 'body management' and includes the development of gross athleticism and fundamental movement skills (balance, control, stability, posture and general fitness). For me, conditioning is all about developing the 'functional capacity' needed to improve and deliver performance. Conditioning has a major role in injury rehabilitation and reconditioning and can contribute to injury reduction.

FUNCTIONAL HYPERTROPHY

We are not talking about getting 'hench' for purely aesthetic reasons. Functional

 Conditioning Cornerstones

Develop or maintain fundamental movement skills and general fitness. Beginners, injury reduction, rehabilitation and reconditioning.
Reps: 10–30 reps
Load: Light (<20% 1RM)
Recovery: <30 seconds
Speed of movement: Slow eccentric, long pause, slow concentric

 Functional Hypertrophy Cornerstones

Develop or maintain optimal levels of muscle size and strength.
Preparation for other training methods.
Reps: 6–15 reps
Load: Medium to heavy (20–80% 1RM)
Recovery: 30–120 seconds
Speed of movement: Slow eccentric, medium pause, slow/medium concentric

hypertrophy is the development of a cross-sectional area (increased muscle size) to achieve a specific performance outcome. Muscle size is a strong predictor of strength and an important prerequisite for strength and power development (phase potentiation). Australian strength and conditioning expert Ian King suggests that hypertrophy training methods can have greater variation, as the primary goal is to create muscle tissue damage and this is achieved through exposure to novel stimuli. When it comes to hypertrophy, variation is good.

MAXIMUM STRENGTH

‘Maximum strength is the maximum amount of force that can be produced during a given movement of unlimited duration.’

Castella and Clews, 1996

In simple terms – load the bar with as much weight as possible and see how much is lifted. Maximum strength is considered to be one of the most important strength qualities. Maximum strength can be subdivided into two types:

1. **Relative** – increasing strength without increasing bodyweight. This approach is important when maximum strength needs to be developed without changes in bodyweight or size.
2. **Absolute** – increasing strength allowing for an increase in bodyweight. Simply put, how much weight can you shift? If I can squat 150kg and you can only squat 100kg, I've got greater absolute strength!

When developing programmes, be aware that maximum strength training should not have the same level of variation seen in other training categories due to the high levels of transfer that are required.

‘When it comes to developing maximal strength you have to train under load. The key is to do this without compromising form.’

Scott Pollock MSc, CSCS, ASCC Senior Strength & Conditioning Coach, English Institute of Sport – British Swimming

Maximum Strength Cornerstones

Develop or maintain higher levels of strength.
Reps: 1–5 (relative) or 4–8 (absolute)
Load: Heavy (>80% 1RM)
Recovery: 120–300 seconds
Speed of movement: Controlled eccentric, short pause, explosive concentric

EXPLOSIVE STRENGTH

Explosive strength is the maximum amount of force that can be produced in a short amount of time and is reliant on the ability of the neuromuscular system to generate very steep increases of force within a split second. Even endurance athletes need to have explosive strength. You only have to watch events like the Tour de France or the London Marathon to see the evidence. For most of the race, the athletes tick along at a steady pace (it's a decent pace, but steady), but at critical moments, when they want to create a breakaway, they will tap into their explosive strength (assuming they've trained it).

‘Power is built on a foundation of strength!! Therefore strength will always be important when trying to be explosive!’

Duncan French PhD, ASCC, CSCS, ASCA-L2. Technical Lead for Strength & Conditioning, English Institute of Sport

Explosive strength can increase by 20–50 per cent in response to heavy resistance training. Factors that have positive impact

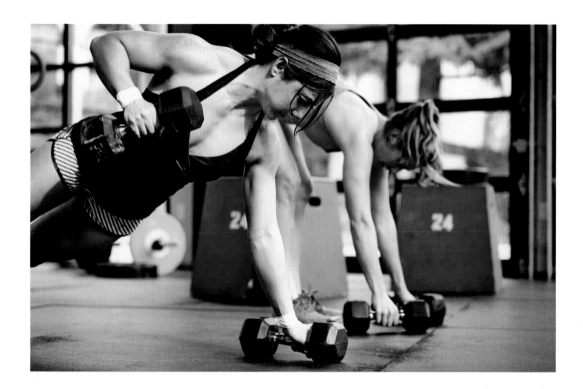

on improvements in explosive strength and expression of power include cross-sectional area (10oz steak instead of 6oz) and increased neural activation (fibre optic broadband instead of dial-up). There are two training methods that can be used to develop explosive strength:

1. **Light** – using lighter loads (20–60% 1RM) and moving them as quickly as possible.
2. **Heavy** – using heavier loads (>80% 1RM) and trying to move them as quickly as possible (explosive maximal 'intent' of external load).

The integration of these different training methods will be dependent on the training requirements of the individual. Each method will work a different portion of the force velocity curve.

 Explosive Strength Cornerstones

Develop or maintain the ability to produce force quickly.

Reps: 6–10 (light) or 1–5 (heavy)
Load: Light (20–60% 1RM) or heavy (>80% 1RM)
Recovery: 30–300 seconds
Speed of movement: Explosive

REACTIVE STRENGTH (SSC)

Reactive strength refers to the ability to effectively use the stretch shortening cycle (SSC) – i.e. the ability to absorb impact (eccentric forces) and explode rapidly from the impact with high levels of force (concentric contraction). Almost all actions require a level of reactive strength (walking, running, hopping, jumping, throwing, hitting, climbing and kicking). Efficient athletes are able to use the elastic properties of tendons and muscles to store and reuse 'elastic energy'. Imagine letting go of a rubber band from a stretched position – it immediately snaps back into its original shape because of its elastic properties.

Reactive Strength (SSC) Cornerstones

Develop ability to move or react quickly.
Reps: 5–20 reps
Load: Light (<10% 1RM)
Recovery: 30–600 seconds
Speed of movement: Explosive

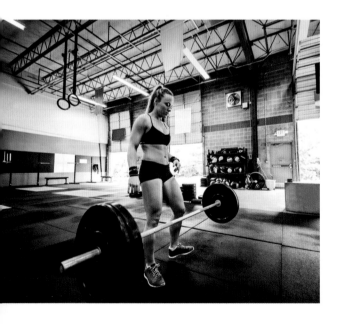

STRENGTH ENDURANCE

Strength endurance refers to the ability to produce force over repeated efforts. Ian King divides strength endurance into three categories:

1. **Continual** – No break or reduction in the attempted expression of strength and the individual is required to minimise the reduction in force over several repeated efforts or throughout the course of a single effort of longer duration.
2. **Intermittent** – Activities that typically have a fixed time frame. Movement is intermittent and requires different expressions of force to be produced over repeated efforts.
3. **Repetitive** – Activities that typically have fixed (longer) time frames. Movement is continuous but force production can change throughout.

Strength Endurance Cornerstones

Maintain a percentage of force with minimal drop off over time.
Reps: 10+ reps
Load: Light (<40% 1RM)
Recovery: 30 seconds
Speed of movement: controlled

◁ A well designed strength programme will unlock your athletic potential

TRAINING METHOD		REPETITIONS	LOAD (% 1RM)	TEMPO			RECOVERY (S)
				ECCCENTRIC	ISOMETRIC	CONCENTRIC	
CONDITIONING		>10	<20%	slow	long	slow	<30
FUNCTIONAL HYPERTROPHY		8-15	20-80%	slow	medium	slow/medium	30-120
MAX STRENGTH	RELATIVE	1-5	>80%	controlled	short	explosive	>120s
	ABSOLUTE	4-8					
EXPLOSIVE POWER		>6	20-60%	fast	none	explosive	30-120
REACTIVE		1-5	>80%	controlled	none	explosive (intent)	>120
CONDITIONING		5-20	<10%	explosive			30-600
STRENGTH ENDURANCE		>15	<40%	controlled			<30s

PROGRAMME DESIGN VARIABLE

Strength programme design matrix

Strength Programme Design Matrix

An understanding of how to apply the correct training modality, the correct volume and intensity and correct timing of each intervention is what every coach and athlete searches for. The strength programme design matrix is a simple reference to help you quickly figure out the key training variables for each strength quality.

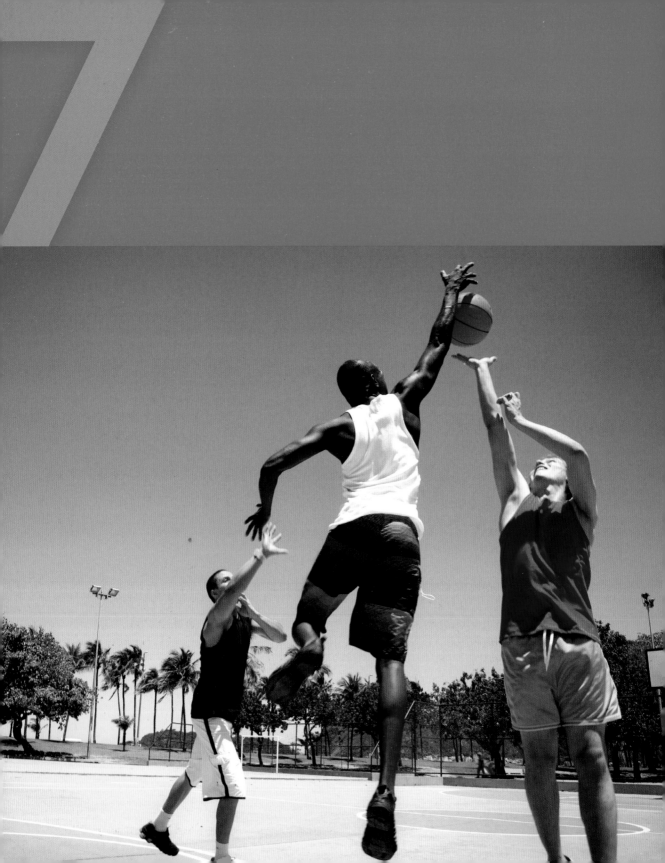

METABOLIC CONDITIONING

■ **Performance ultimately depends on the capacity** to produce power for the duration of an event, and on the efficiency with which that energy is translated into movement. (Peter Snell, 800 & 1500m Gold Medallist, 1964 Olympics)

Metabolic conditioning is a term used to describe conditioning exercises intended to increase the storage and delivery of energy for any activity. The ability to resist fatigue is multifactorial and linked to efficiency and coordination of our body systems: cardiovascular, metabolic and nervous. Modern training methods recognise the importance of developing training programmes that improve both central and peripheral adaptations, while the ultimate goal of metabolic conditioning is to develop the ability to produce effort with minimal drop in performance. Vern Gambetta makes a valid point in his book *Athletic Development: The Art & Science of Functional Sports Conditioning* when he says that while an 'aerobic' base is important for endurance-based athletes, the real goal for the majority of the population is to develop a strong foundation of general fitness '*work capacity*' – the ability to tolerate a workload and recover from it.

‘Anxiety is a key training tool with my athletes, if they're not anxious about the session planned then it's not training – it's exercise. The work capacity demands of MetCon both physically and mentally are ideal for this.’

Darren Roberts High Performance Manager, Harris and Ross Healthcare

When you exercise you will challenge the metabolic, neuromuscular and musculoskeletal systems. Exactly what proportion of each of those systems is called into play depends largely on the programme design. But before we tackle the more traditional training concepts surrounding programme design, we need to get to grips with some of the fundamental physiology. It will get a bit sciency, but stick with it.

When we talk about developing the metabolic system, we are referring to three distinct yet closely related integrated biochemical processes:

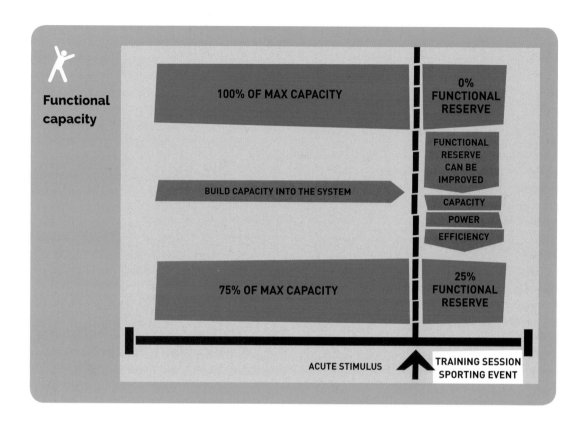

1. Splitting of the stored phosphagens
2. Anaerobic breakdown of carbohydrate
3. Aerobic breakdown of carbohydrates and fats

Bioenergetics – Energy Systems

All energy is derived from the 'high energy' molecule – ATP (Adenosine Triphosphate). ATP has three phosphate molecules attached to it by high-energy chemical bonds. When a bond is broken, energy is released and used by the muscle to produce work.

Your ability to regenerate ATP dictates performance potential. ATP is the primary energy currency of the cell and is used for a wide and diverse range of functions, including hormone production, muscle contractions, generating new body tissue, nerve conduction, repairing damaged tissue, and digesting and processing food. In fact, it's a pretty complex molecule that plays a vital role in numerous biological reactions that take place in the body.

There are three ways to generate energy for the muscles so that they can perform exercise:

1. ATP-PC
2. Anaerobic
3. Aerobic

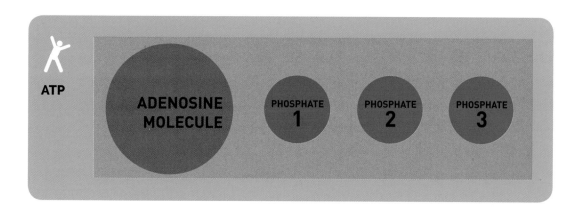

ATP

ADENOSINE MOLECULE

PHOSPHATE 1

PHOSPHATE 2

PHOSPHATE 3

ATP-PC | Anaerobic | Aerobic

1. ATP-PC SYSTEM (IMMEDIATE)

The ATP-PC system provides instant energy. When your body needs instant energy (e.g. sprinting for the bus), the phosphates are split

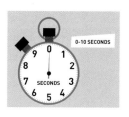

0-10 SECONDS

from the ATP molecule to provide energy (1–4 seconds). Once the energy has been released for mechanical work by the muscle, phosphocreatine (PC), another high-energy compound, can be used to 'reboot' the energy supply, adding the potential for another 5–10 seconds of energy. As with the levels of ATP stored in the cell, there is an extremely limited supply of PC. Once this energy source has been exhausted, the body needs to find other ways to resupply the muscle with ATP. If you've not caught the bus by the time, you've exhausted your immediate energy supply and the chances are you'll be walking to work!

2. ANAEROBIC SYSTEM (SHORT)

The anaerobic system produces ATP at a fast rate. There are fewer chemical steps than in the aerobic system and the anaerobic system

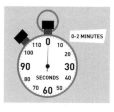

0-2 MINUTES

is used to produce energy rapidly for large (high-intensity) but short-term power outputs. This time, the fuel comes in the form of carbohydrate (*glucose* – blood, or *glycogen* – muscle/liver) and different chemical pathways are used to generate the energy needed. The total amount of energy the anaerobic system can produce is limited, due to the high levels of lactic acid that result from the chemical reactions taking place to produce ATP. The anaerobic system can supply enough energy for another 60–120 seconds of work; once depleted, the body experiences rapid power reduction and a drop in speed of movement.

3. AEROBIC SYSTEM (LONG)

The aerobic energy system produces ATP at a much slower rate than anaerobic metabolism for low–moderate intensity and long-duration 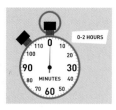 activities. The aerobic system is oxygen-dependent (needs oxygen to be delivered to the lungs, transferred into the blood and transported to the working muscles) and produces large amounts of energy (most ATP per given substrate) but it uses more chemical reactions and takes longer. The aerobic system breaks down carbohydrate and fat and even protein to produce ATP. The aerobic system can supply enough energy for up to 2 hours of work.

THE ENERGY SYSTEM CONTINUUM

The contribution from each energy system varies according to the intensity and duration of the activity and the body's fuel supply. All of the systems are working but the intensity and duration of the effort will dictate the proportionate contribution. The energy system operates using 'energy autoselect' – the choice of energy system is dictated by the demand for ATP. If the demand for energy is high and rapid, anaerobic systems will predominantly be used for energy production; if it is low and slow, aerobic systems will predominantly be used.

Metabolic Conditioning For Performance Enhancement

‘*Metabolic conditioning can be made interesting, varied and more effective through choosing different modalities and parameters.*’

Pete McKnight BSc, CSCS, ASCC. Chairman of the UKSCA. Strength & Conditioning Coach, French Ski Team

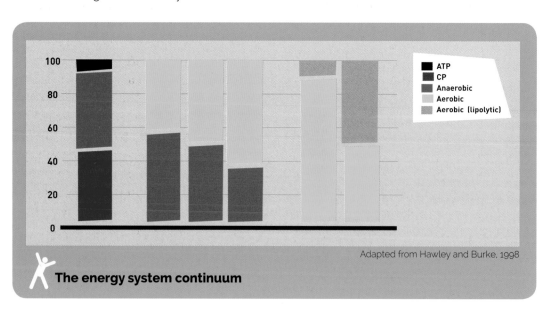

Adapted from Hawley and Burke, 1998

The energy system continuum

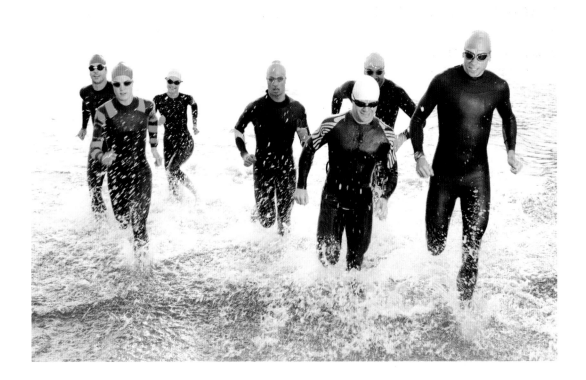

Get ready to shift your mindset and embrace a more effective approach to metabolic conditioning. The days of the slow steady run could be well and truly over!

Historically, endurance training has focused on the central adaptations (cardiovascular) and paid scant attention to peripheral adaptations (neuromuscular). Experts such as the late Mel Siff have been telling us for decades that the development of endurance is closely linked with the musculoskeletal system but it has largely fallen on deaf ears, until recently. Metabolic conditioning is more complex than simply trying to develop lungs like dustbin liners. The physiological responses of any session will be affected by the respective contribution of the three metabolic processes (central adaptations) and the musculoskeletal strain (peripheral adaptations).

Modern training paradigms recognise the importance of developing training programmes that improve both central and peripheral adaptations. It's no longer a simple case of heading out for a slow run or long bike ride. Remember, it's the musculoskeletal system that drives the body. We now recognise that, when programmed properly, we can develop our metabolic systems using a wide range of training interventions, including strength training. Research shows that both high-intensity interval training and a more traditional volume-based approach using lower training intensities can effectively improve cardiac and skeletal muscle metabolic function. The ultimate aim of metabolic conditioning should be to develop the ability to produce effort with minimal drop off. We can challenge the system by running, swimming, rowing, cycling and even lifting!

Better results in less time is always our motto at Results Fitness. For this reason our Metabolic Conditioning workouts include heart rate monitors, multiple planes of motion, load using kettlebells and sand bags among other tools and all seven movements of the human body (squat, bend, push, pull, twist, single-leg balance, lunge). To get your body to change you have to put a demand on it that it is not used to. For most people conditioning workouts need to go beyond a jog on the treadmill.

Rachel Cosgrove CSCS, BS Physiology, 2012 IDEA Personal Trainer of the Year. Owner of Results Fitness and Results Fitness University

Conventional training models work on a 'results by volume' approach, developing an 'aerobic base' using general aerobic (slow and steady) conditioning sessions. While this may still be an appropriate method to use during the early stages of training for short periods of time, it has limitations. The problem with this type of training is twofold: it's not particularly efficient (sessions are long and tedious) and there's an increased risk of chronic 'overuse' injuries (you're pounding the streets for longer and exposing your body to the same movement over and over again).

REVERSE PERIODISATION

There is an alternative approach that is often a more effective training method. Reverse periodisation is a training concept based on maintaining intensity closer to that of the demands of the activity. It makes intuitive sense, particularly when we consider function and specificity, as discussed earlier in the book. As you progress through training the volume is increased, while still maintaining training intensity. This training method has gathered pace since its inception back in the 1980s and has been applied successfully by many of the world's leading coaches.

The ultimate outcome is that, by training at a higher intensity with lower volumes, your body will begin to adapt and be capable of

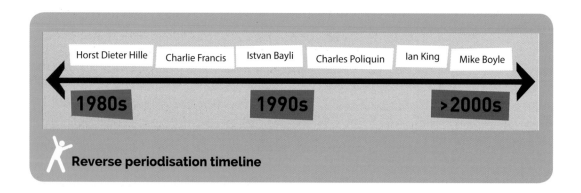

Horst Dieter Hille Charlie Francis Istvan Bayli Charles Poliquin Ian King Mike Boyle

1980s 1990s >2000s

Reverse periodisation timeline

Two athletes want to run a half-marathon in 1 hour 45 minutes. That means they will need to run at an 8:01 minutes per mile pace. At the moment, neither athlete can maintain that pace for more than 2 miles. Traditional periodisation would suggest that athlete A starts his training by developing an aerobic base using long, slow, steady efforts at below race pace. Running at a tempo slower than race pace is relatively easy and athlete A is able to build up some longer

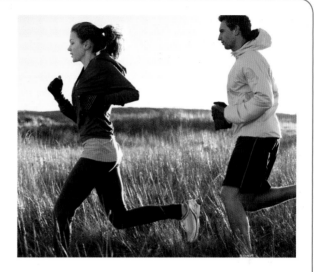

runs, even though they are at a slower pace. Once the base level of aerobic fitness has been developed, he will start to reduce the overall volume of training and increase the intensity (pace), so that he is eventually able to complete the distance at the desired pace. This is where the problems start. The large volume of slow steady running means that the body has adapted specifically to running slow and steady. Remember, it's not just about developing central adaptations; we need to consider peripheral adaptations too. Try running at two different paces. I guarantee that running at a 9:30/mile pace compared to an 8:01/mile pace will feel different. You will challenge the metabolic, neuromuscular and musculoskeletal systems differently. We have to remember that the exact proportion of each of those systems that is called into play depends largely on the programme design. It's tough to switch from slow and steady to fast and furious.

Athlete B opts for the reverse periodisation strategy and starts off working on repeated efforts over a distance at which he can maintain race pace. Volume is then gradually increased so that the athlete eventually builds up his specific endurance capacity to be able to cope with the full half-marathon distance at race pace. Running at race pace from day one of training will develop the metabolic, neuromuscular and musculoskeletal demands that will be needed on race day right from the get go, rather than waiting to 'switch' to race pace halfway through the training programme.

Both athletes can get to the same end point, but in my opinion Athlete B has taken the smarter option. While reverse periodisation is often my preferred approach when working with athletes, deconditioned or injured individuals may find that a more traditional approach is more appropriate when returning to fitness.

tolerating training at appropriate intensities right from day one. You will always be training in a manner that elicits specific central and peripheral adaptations for a given training intensity and then it's a case of simply cranking up the training volume.

Athlete B may approach his training for the race progression using the three steps outlined below:

Step#1: Power

Training will comprise shorter efforts with reduced recovery to flood the body with lactate and develop the anaerobic pathways. The aim of this phase is to develop the ability to produce high levels of intense work with minimal drop in performance within the time

frame of the specific endurance sub-quality (amount of energy produced per unit of time). This type of training develops the ability to tolerate accumulation of lactate and will have an impact on the musculoskeletal system.

Step #2: Capacity

Training will typically take the shape of longer-duration efforts aimed at ensuring that you have a good level of underpinning aerobic endurance. This is all about increasing the size of the tank to produce work with minimal diminishment within the time frame of a specific endurance sub-quality (either over a long period of time, or repetitively). Capacity is relevant at both ends of the time frame within each sub-quality, or at any time within the time frame in a repetitive situation.

Step #3: Efficiency

This type of training recognises the need to have a level of movement efficiency and robustness to complete more 'task specific' training (acceleration, deceleration, change of direction, jumping, hopping, big lifts). This form of training develops both central and peripheral adaptations from an aerobic and anaerobic standpoint but now you are throwing a significant mechanical load into the training session. Optimal use of available energy (metabolic and mechanical) allows you to work at a greater percentage of maximum with less energy cost (coordination, agility, vision, reflexes, strength). Efficiency is relevant at both ends of the time frame within each sub-quality.

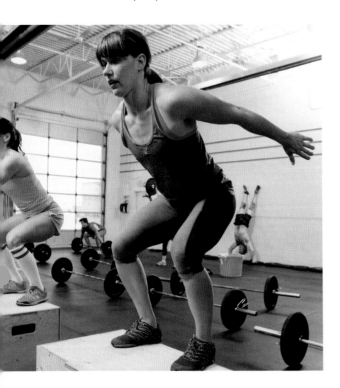

◁ Become an efficient mover

Metabolic Conditioning Strategies

In the table below I've taken three broad training strategies and provided a summary to give you an idea of the most suitable approach to adopt for your training. If your goal is simply to develop some base fitness, using a continuous strategy is going to be a good option for you. It's suitable for developing work capacity (size of the tank) and is more suited to traditional exercise modalities, such as running and cycling. If, however, you are looking for a workout that is going to challenge both the central and peripheral systems, include some interval-based training in your programme.

This type of training is really good for non-endurance-based events and will suit you if you are looking to work over shorter efforts using non-traditional training methods such as strength training.

METABOLIC CONDITIONING – SUB-QUALITIES

Several sub-qualities of metabolic conditioning exist and the performance outcome and your fitness profile will determine the relevance and effectiveness of each sub-quality as part of an integrated performance conditioning programme. In this table I've provided an overview of training prescriptions for each sub-quality.

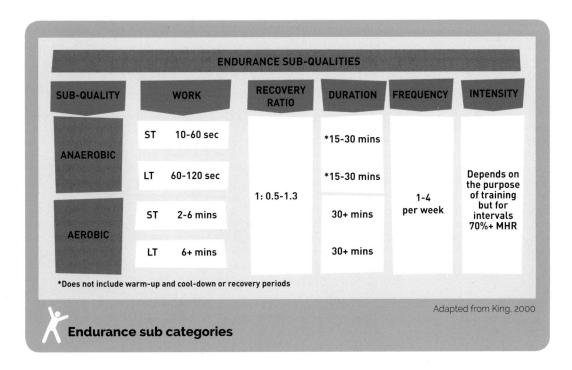

ENDURANCE SUB-QUALITIES

SUB-QUALITY	WORK		RECOVERY RATIO	DURATION	FREQUENCY	INTENSITY
ANAEROBIC	ST	10-60 sec		*15-30 mins		
	LT	60-120 sec		*15-30 mins		Depends on the purpose of training but for intervals 70%+ MHR
	ST	2-6 mins	1: 0.5-1.3	30+ mins	1-4 per week	
AEROBIC	LT	6+ mins		30+ mins		

*Does not include warm-up and cool-down or recovery periods

Adapted from King, 2000

Endurance sub categories

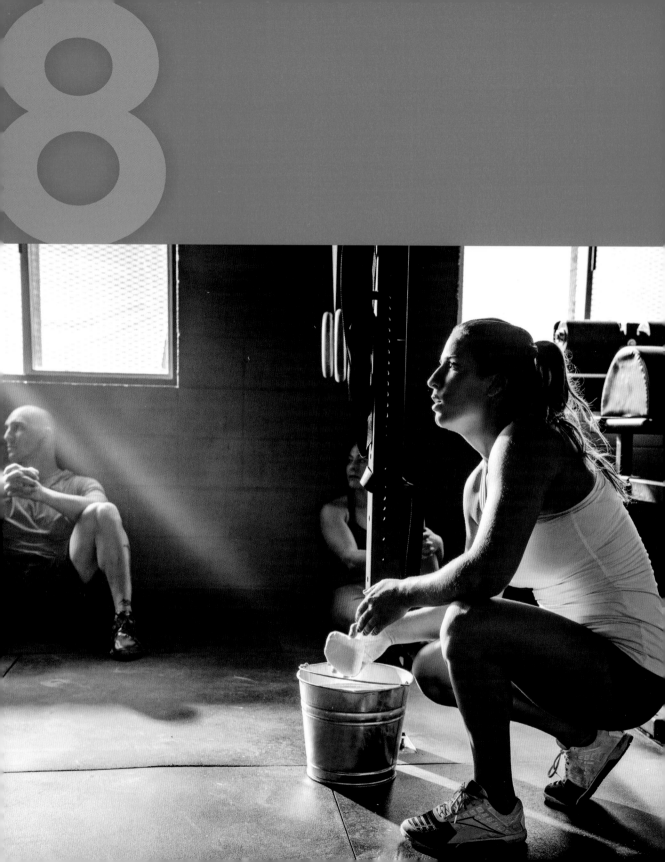

8

RECOVERY AND REGENERATION

■ **If you are reading this book** it's probably because you love to keep fit and want to optimise your training, but how can you push yourself in training without tipping your body over the edge? How can you train hard without falling apart? The answer is one of the simplest yet most neglected training principles – recovery and regeneration.

> *I have always thought recovery and regeneration is about getting all the performance fundamentals optimised first and foremost.*
>
> **Grant Downie** OBE, MCSP HCPC. Head of Performance, Manchester City FC Academy

Training and competing for an event or simply hitting the gym on a regular basis places significant demands on your body. Running a marathon, taking part in an adventure race or playing for your local football team for the season can sometimes push your body and mind to the limit. This is just the event itself; combine that with a hectic home and social life and you had better make sure you are able to adapt to the demands that you are placing on your body. If you cannot adapt to and cope with the physical and mental requirements of training, competition and the game of life, you will quickly become exhausted.

Training creates a physiological stress on your body and it disturbs homeostasis at a cellular level. A tough training session or hard game can result in low-grade systemic inflammatory responses. These responses can sometimes stick around in your body for up to 5 days and during this time your immune system can be impaired, leaving you more susceptible to infections and illness.

> Failure to recover sufficiently from the continuous demands and stress of life, training and competition can lead to a cycle of impaired performance and accumulated fatigue.

The ability of your body to regain its physiological balance is dependent on its ability to recover. To encourage adaptation to training, it is important to plan recovery activities that reduce residual fatigue. Planned periods of recovery and regeneration provide an opportunity for training-based adaptations to take place, enabling the body to cope with future training sessions.

This is not a new concept – the scientific community has been aware of its importance since the 1940s and it should be the very cornerstone of your integrated performance conditioning programme. The General Adaptation Syndrome (GAS) developed by Hans Selye in the 1940s established that there must be a period of low-intensity training or complete recovery following periods of intense training. The three phases of the GAS play a pivotal role in our understanding of recovery and regeneration.

Progressive Overload

Work alone is not enough to produce the best results. Your body needs time to adapt to training.

To encourage adaptation to training, it is important to plan recovery activities that reduce residual fatigue. The sooner you recover from fatigue, the fresher you will be when you complete your next training session and the better your chance of improving. Remember, training is designed to progressively overload the body systems and fuel stores and it must be applied carefully to improve performance.

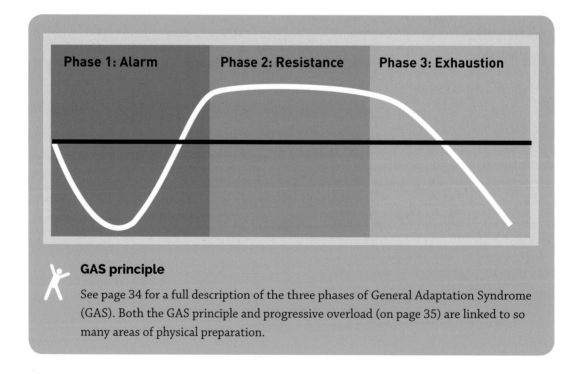

Phase 1: Alarm   **Phase 2: Resistance**   **Phase 3: Exhaustion**

GAS principle

See page 34 for a full description of the three phases of General Adaptation Syndrome (GAS). Both the GAS principle and progressive overload (on page 35) are linked to so many areas of physical preparation.

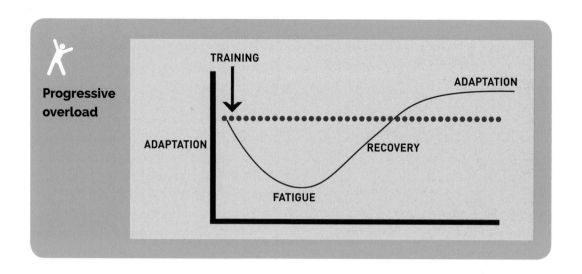

Progressive overload

If the training stress is inadequate to overload the physiological system, no adaptations will occur. If the workload is too great (applied too quickly, performed too often without adequate rest), fatigue follows and the performance will be reduced.

FATIGUE CONTINUUM

When you complete an intense period of training (or even a single training session), you will become fatigued – it's inevitable. You may even notice a short-term drop in performance. This is a normal function of training and is termed Functional Overreaching (FO):

- Short-term fatigue experienced during heavy training periods
- Physical performance may temporarily be reduced
- A short period of recovery (days–weeks) results in supercompensation and increased physical capacity.

If you extend the period of heavy training with inadequate recovery, your physical performance(s) plateau and chronic fatigue results in a sustained reduction in physical capacity. This is far from ideal and is known as Non-Functional Overreaching (NFO):

- Chronic fatigue results in a sustained reduction in physical capacity
- Physical performance(s) plateau
- A longer period of recovery (weeks–months) is required in order to return to normal functioning

Overtraining Syndrome (OTS) is the term given to long-term fatigue experienced during sustained periods of heavy training. This can be a serious problem caused by a significant and prolonged imbalance between training and recovery, resulting in reduced performance, injury, illness and chronic maladaptations.

> *'Formula 1, the fastest sport on earth, is won by those who learn how to take pit stops most effectively. The same principles apply to humans.'*

Professor Damian Hughes Professor of Organisational Psychology and Change, Manchester Metropolitan University

WHAT IS FATIGUE?

Fatigue is multifactorial – depending on the type of training or competition stimulus, you will experience a number of different forms of fatigue as a result of training and competition.

Metabolic

Typically results from high-volume training with repeated workloads (aerobic/anaerobic conditioning) and multiple training sessions throughout the day, resulting in depleted energy stores.

Tissue damage

If you compete in contact sports, you'll be susceptible to fatigue resulting from tissue damage (dead legs, bruising etc). Plyometric training can also create high levels of muscle damage due to the eccentric loading patterns.

Neurological

The peripheral nervous system is fatigued as a result of high-intensity training and resistance training (strength and power development). Speed work and skill-based sessions where new training techniques are introduced can also result in neurological fatigue.

Psychological

Training monotony can lead to central nervous system (CNS) fatigue. Heavy competition and training periods as well as high-pressure situations can take their toll on your ability to recovery sufficiently. It is also important that you recognise the impact that your lifestyle can have on your ability to train and compete (stressful job, relationship problems, exam periods etc) and how emotionally draining this can be.

Environmental

Environmental conditions such as heat, cold and altitude can all cause fatigue. Travel (local, national, international) and time differences can also play a role in fatigue and shouldn't be overlooked.

Recovery Strategies

Despite an increased understanding of the importance of recovery and regeneration, we are still faced with a huge variety of interventions, which can become extremely confusing. Recovery interventions can be broken down into two broad categories:

1. **Prophylactic** – recovery interventions that can be put in place prior to training. *Nutrition, supplementation, compression garments, prior eccentric activity, flexibility and mobility, reactive programming.*
2. **Therapeutic** – recovery interventions that are used after training. *Active and passive rest, pool-based therapy, massage therapy, electrotherapies, hydrotherapies, anti-inflammatory drugs and cryotherapy.*

THE RECOVERY PYRAMID

Just as there are different types of fatigue, there is also a number of options available when it comes to recovery. It's easy to get carried away with all the latest fads and trends such as compression clothing and ice baths while forgetting about the basics such as sleep and nutrition. The recovery pyramid presents a more structured and balanced approach to recovery and regeneration. Let's take a closer look at some of the recovery and regeneration strategies that are available to you.

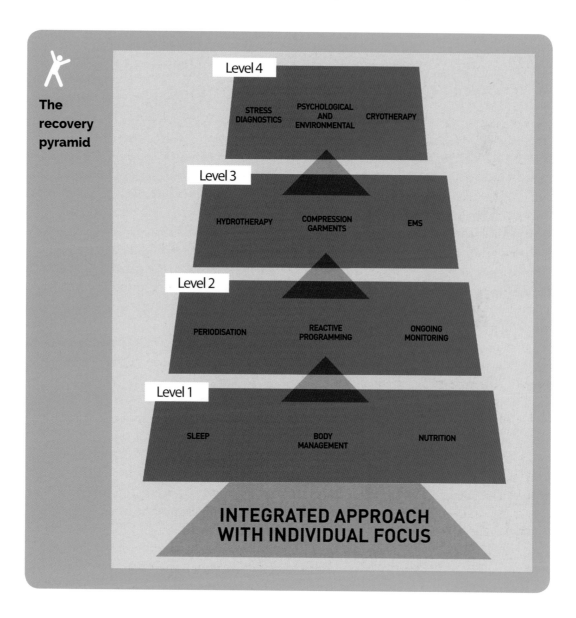

The recovery pyramid

Level 4

STRESS DIAGNOSTICS — PSYCHOLOGICAL AND ENVIRONMENTAL — CRYOTHERAPY

Level 3

HYDROTHERAPY — COMPRESSION GARMENTS — EMS

Level 2

PERIODISATION — REACTIVE PROGRAMMING — ONGOING MONITORING

Level 1

SLEEP — BODY MANAGEMENT — NUTRITION

INTEGRATED APPROACH WITH INDIVIDUAL FOCUS

"Unless you get the basic pillars of recovery right (sleep, nutrition, hydration), the benefits to be gained from any other modalities, no matter how hi-tech, will be minimal."

Chris Barnes MSc, BSc, CSci. Head of Sports Science, West Bromwich Albion FC

Sleep

Sleep is one of the most important forms of rest and provides time for you to adapt to the physical and mental demands of training. Studies have shown that as little as 30–36 hours of sleep deprivation can result in a loss of performance (physical, mental). Those hours don't all have to occur at the same time, they can be accumulated over a period of time. Cutting back on your sleep over the course of a week could push you into sleep debt.

Nutrition (refuelling and rehydration)

Nutrition is one of the cornerstones of a comprehensive recovery and regeneration strategy and can be strategically used to optimise training and performance. A solid approach to refuelling and rehydrating will have a positive impact on your response to exercise in terms of hormone control and muscle function. Get the basics right:

1. Eat regularly
2. Go easy on sugars and processed food
3. Eat fruit and vegetables
4. Drink plenty of water (2.5 litres per day)

Body Management (passive and active rest)

Forms of passive rest include reading, listening to music, watching a film etc. Active rest such as walking, cross-training and flexibility/mobility training are also beneficial to your overall recovery.

"Sleep, nutrition and hydration are all obviously important for recovery – but the forgotten factor is social time with family and friends. The mind needs a break just like the body does."

Darren Roberts. High Performance Manager, Harris and Ross Healthcare

Massage

There is an increasing use of massage in the recovery strategies of many high-performance athletes and it's increasingly becoming a mainstream approach for recreational athletes and weekend warriors too. Physiological benefits of massage may include: increased blood flow; enhanced oxygen and nutrient delivery to fatigued muscles; increased removal of lactic acid; warming and stretching of soft tissues, increasing flexibility and the removal of micro trauma, knots and adhesions. The psychological benefits of massage should not be underestimated and may include improved mood state, increased relaxation and feeling less fatigued. Massage can also improve your body awareness.

Cool Down

The 'cool-down' is a group of exercises performed immediately after training to provide a period of adjustment between exercise and rest. It's probably the most neglected part of a training session but you omit it at your peril. Implementing a proper cool-down will improve muscular relaxation, remove waste products,

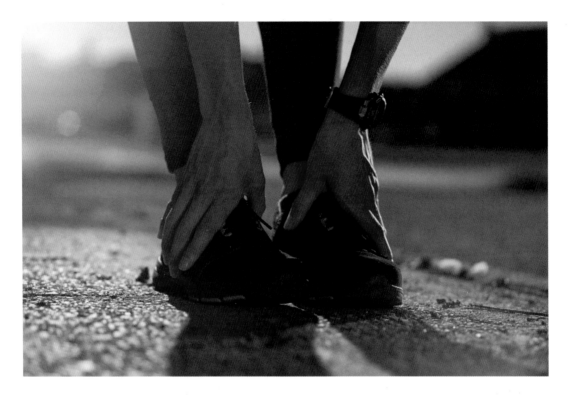

reduce muscular soreness and bring the cardiovascular system back to rest.

Flexibility and Mobility

Flexibility and mobility training is possibly the most forgotten, misunderstood and misapplied aspect of recovery and regeneration. Increased flexibility and mobility will allow you to move your limbs smoothly and easily through an unrestricted, pain-free range of motion and a regenerative flexibility and mobility session is a great way to recover physically and mentally from training and competition.

Periodisation

Pioneers such as Verkhoshansky, Matveyev, Zatsiorsky, Nadori, Bompa, Bondarchuk and Balyi have established periodisation as one of the fundamental components of any training programme. Your ability to recover from training and competition will be enhanced through the use of a well-planned training programme, which allows time to recover from the training being undertaken.

 Reactive Programming

Once you have a plan, accept that there will be times when you need to deviate from it in order to recover! The ability for you to react to a given situation is crucial to the success of the programme. If you feel shattered, there is little point training for the sake of sticking to the programme.

Ongoing Monitoring

Regular monitoring can provide 'early warnings' that a recovery intervention is required. A simple training diary or recovery diary can provide an insight into how you are adapting to training and areas that can be improved.

	POSSIBLE POINTS	DAY OF THE WEEK						
		M	T	W	T	F	S	S
NUTRITION	8							
Breakfast	1							
Lunch	2							
Dinner	2							
Pre-workout Snack	1							
Post-exercise carb refuelling within 60 minutes. Recommended 1.0 to 1.5g per kg of bodyweight	2							
HYDRATION	2							
Pre-exercise urine: clear or light	1							
Post-exercise urine: clear or light	1							
SLEEP AND REST	4							
8 hours of restful sleep	3							
Nap during the day	1							
RELAXATION AND EMOTIONAL STATUS	3							
No daily psycho-social stress	1							
Fully relaxed 60 minutes Post-workout or 30 minutes of feet-up relaxation post workout	2							
FLEXIBILITY/MOBILITY/COOL-DOWN	3							
Adequate cool-down after exercise	2							
Flexibility/Mobility for at least 10 minutes	1							
TOTAL*	20							

Hydrotherapies

- **Pool Session:** Swimming pools provide an excellent environment in which to conduct a recovery session. Water provides buoyancy and resistance properties that allow you to complete training with minimal impact on the body. Many experts recommend completing a 20-minute pool-based recovery session the day after a heavy training session or competition.

- **Contrast Bathing:** Alternating hot and cold showers/baths could provide an increase in blood flow to the working muscles, accelerating the removal of metabolic by-products. Researchers also suggest that contrast bathing could stimulate the nervous system and help to increase arousal.

- **Cold Baths:** Cold baths have primarily been used for their pain-relieving properties.

More recently, the thinking behind this one is that when you plunge your body into a bath full of icy cold water, vasoconstriction will kick in and the blood will be drained away from the muscles that have been working (removing lactic acid). When you get out of the bath, the capillaries dilate and 'new' blood flows back to the muscles, bringing with it oxygen, which helps the functioning of the cells. Research seems to support the use of ice baths and has shown that cold water immersion can improve muscle function, reduce muscle damage and decrease soreness associated with delayed onset muscle soreness (DOMS).

Compression Garments

Next time your favourite football or rugby team take to the pitch, check out what they are wearing beneath their shirts, shorts and socks. Chances are it will be something a little more sophisticated than a vest – it's more likely to be a compression garment. This is one of the latest boom businesses in terms of recovery, and leading sports apparel manufacturers are producing garments with 'compression qualities'. Heavy training can cause muscle damage resulting in soreness, swelling, pain and impaired athletic performance. Scientific research has indicated that external compression can be an effective treatment that minimises swelling and improves the alignment and mobility of scar tissue following eccentric damage and DOMS.

Electrical Muscle Stimulation (EMS)

Electrical muscle stimulation (EMS), also known as neuromuscular electrical stimulation (NMES) or electromyostimulation, has received increasing attention in recent years. It is believed that it can help to speed up the muscle recovery process through increased venous circulation for the accelerated removal of metabolic waste immediately after exercise, reducing DOMS within 24 hours, for accelerated muscle recovery.

 Stress Diagnostics

Modern technology can help you to take an 'inside look' at how your body is functioning. Various systems are available and will measure a range of paramaters such as heart rate variability (HRV) to provide objective data relating to training, recovery and sleep, allowing you to make informed decisions about your training.

Psychological and Environmental

Floatation tanks (restricted environmental stimulation therapy), sleep pods etc can provide an environment with minimal stimulation. Reducing the amount of stimulation to the brain allows you to focus more effectively on relaxing and becoming emotionally calm. Potential mechanisms include:

- Decreased production of cortisol, ACTH, lactic acid and adrenaline
- Increased production of endorphins (pain-reducing substances released by the hypothalamus and pituitary gland)

Cryotherapy

Whole-body cryotherapy (WBC) consists of exposure to very cold air that is maintained at 110–140°C in temperature-controlled cryochambers, generally for 2–4 minutes for 1–2 sessions per day (20–40 exposures in total). WBC is used to relieve pain and inflammatory symptoms. It has gained wider acceptance as a way of improving recovery from muscle injury.

> Recovery and regeneration is a key component of an integrated performance conditioning programme. If we are not careful, the basics are going to be forgotten and everyone will focus on the latest trend. With this in mind, you would be well advised to think about the fundamental principles relating to training and recovery in order to make an informed decision about which recovery method is the most suitable.

 Recovery and Regeneration Essentials

- Training should be designed to progressively overload the body's systems and fuel stores.
- Fatigue has various forms (metabolic, tissue damage, neurological, environmental, psychological).
- Remember the basics, use the recovery pyramid and put the cornertones in place first. Eat well and get adequate rest; the fancy stuff can come later.

RECOVERY AND REGENERATION MATRIX

Recovery and regeneration is not a one-size-fits-all approach. It is a process and should form the cornerstone of a structured training programme so that you can attain the maximal possible physiological adaptations while reducing the risk of residual fatigue, which may result in illness or injury. Each component of the recovery pyramid is an essential 'building block'; the mortar that holds the blocks together is your ability to apply the concepts described in this section using an integrated approach with an individual focus. While it's not an exact science, the recovery and regeneration matrix will give you a head start on which recovery strategy may be the most appropriate for any given type of fatigue. Remember, get the basics established first before you try to get too clever.

Periodisation of Recovery Strategies

Does the use of recovery and regeneration strategies offer short-term benefits at the expense of long-term adaptation? It is worth remembering that if the training stress is inadequate to overload the physiological system, then no adaptations will occur. It is important that you recognise that immediate use of recovery and regeneration strategies can reduce the natural ability of the body to restore itself and promote adaptation. If you continue to use the same type of recovery and regeneration strategy, you may actually decrease the recuperative effect. Experts

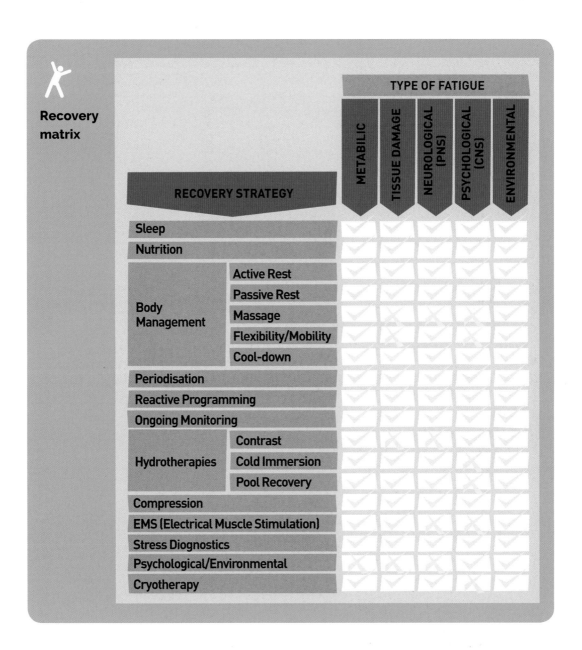

Recovery matrix

recommend that the same recovery strategy should not be applied more than once or twice a week in the same form. When developing a recovery and regeneration strategy, you should consider the same fundamental principles that you apply to training programme design (accommodation, progressive overload, use/disuse).

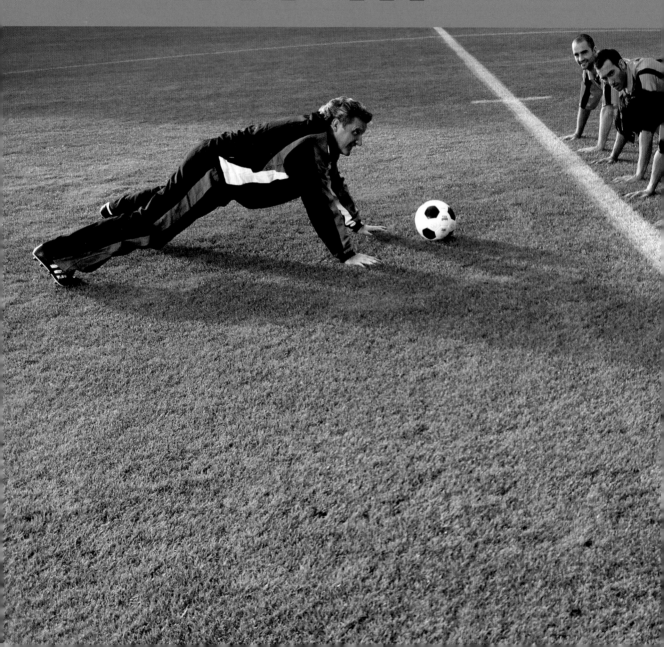

PART III

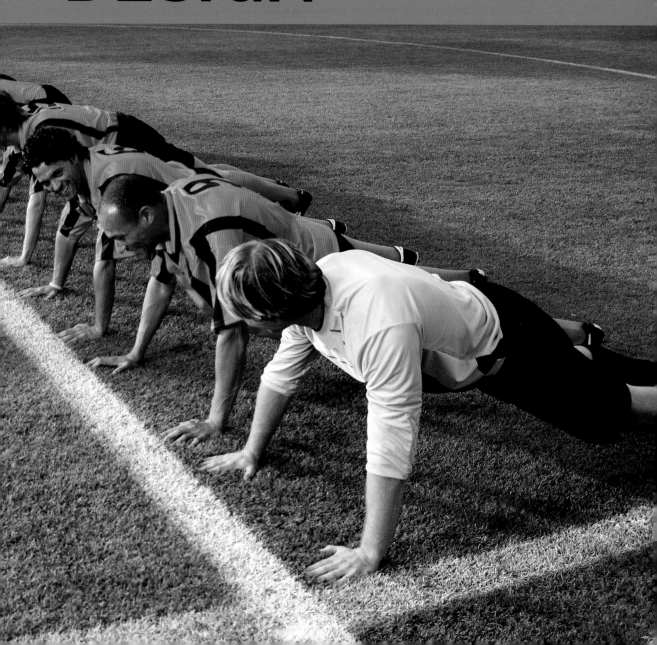

PROGRAMME DESIGN

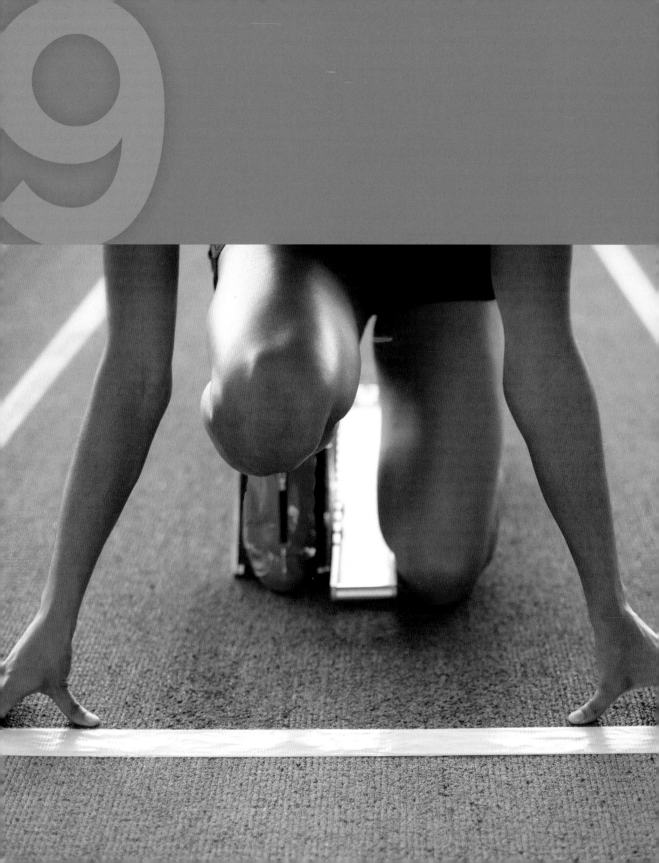

9

EFFECTIVE PROGRAMME DESIGN

■ **If you've got this far, you should be pretty excited** about starting to implement some of the training strategies that we've covered throughout the book.

The problem is that at the moment you've got a bunch of great ideas and basic frameworks to work from but no real understanding of how to bring it all together. You're not alone, there are a lot of professional coaches and athletes who struggle to pull all of their good ideas together in one coherent programme. In this section, I'll give you the essential tools that will allow you to develop your own training programme.

'The longer I coach, the more I realise that optimum performance is nothing to do with fancy training methods or new gimmicks. There truly is nothing new under the sun. The best performers are those who take the same information that everybody else has, then who organise it and apply it in the most efficient manner possible. Great programme design is the foundation of this success.'

Keir Wenham-Flatt MSc, CSCS. Lead strength coach, Los Pumas Argentina

Producing an integrated performance conditioning programme is a bit like learning to cook. At the moment you have all of your ingredients laid out in front of you but you've only just learned the difference between cucumber and couscous. You could try to make a meal but it would be pretty nasty! Most fitness books will give you basic recipes to follow and this book is no exception. There are some core programme templates (recipes) for you to follow at the back of the book. But that's not where we will leave it, because while that may help to get you started, you'll probably want to go on to develop your own individualised programme.

In addition to the programme templates, I'm going to share with you the essential principles of programme design. This is going to be programme design stripped back to the fundamentals. I'll show you how to manipulate training variables and select and sequence exercises and sessions effectively to develop fully integrated performance conditioning programmes. At the end of the section you'll get a programme design checklist that will allow you to develop effectively your own weekly and monthly training programmes. These are the cornerstones of my programme design principles; other techniques and strategies may come and go, but these elements form the foundations on which all my programmes are built.

Understanding some of the key principles allows you to create your own programmes, which are a roadmap for success and achieving your goals.

Pete McKnight BSc, CSCS, ASCC. Chairman of the UKSCA. Strength & Conditioning Coach, French Ski Team

To achieve consistent performance outcomes, you must be able to design an integrated training programme that addresses your individual needs. While programme design

The Goldilocks Principle

Develop a training programme that is 'just right'.

is a complex subject, we can cut through a lot of the complexity if we take a leaf out of Goldilocks' book.

Each bear had their own bowl of porridge, chair and bed. After testing each of the three, Goldilocks determined that one was always too much at one extreme (too hot, too large, etc), one was too much at the opposite extreme (too cold, too small, etc), and one was 'just right'. Fitness coaches and athletes often fall into the trap of producing and following programmes that are either 'too hot' or 'too cold'. If you develop your programme design skills, you will be able to produce programmes that are 'just right'.

Planning

Programme design involves making use of a purposeful system or plan to achieve a specific goal.

Clark & Lucett. 2010

At the very beginning of this book, I made a point of highlighting the importance of working to a plan that is related to a task or performance outcome. If you don't have a training plan linked to a performance outcome then there *is* no plan to your training and you are ultimately just 'doing work', treading the same path but always ending up back at the same point. Remember the words of renowned strength and conditioning coach Vern Gambetta: he simply said 'everyone should train with a purpose'.

Our desire for control is so powerful and the feeling of being in control so rewarding, that

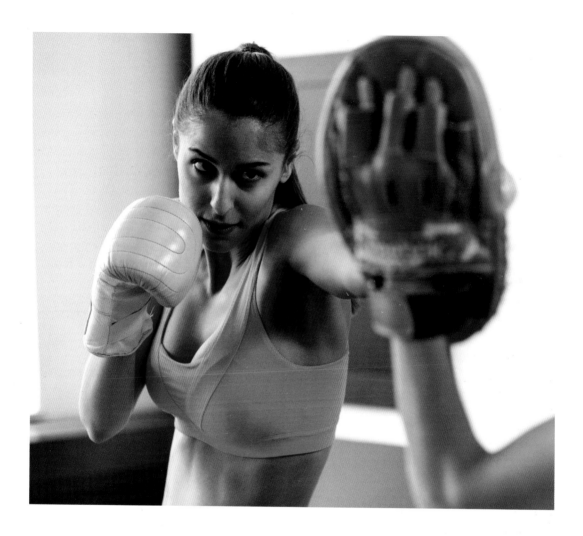

we often act as though we are controlling the uncontrollable. For instance, people feel more certain that they will win the lottery if they can control the numbers they choose on the tickets and feel more confident they will win a dice toss if they can throw the dice themselves. Shaping a programme increases engagement and effectiveness.

Professor Damian Hughes Professor of Organisational Psychology and Change, Manchester Metropolitan University

 Why develop a structured programme?

- Structure training in order to ensure improvement
- Improve general and specific areas
- Peak for major goals
- Prevent overtraining
- Injury reduction

Poor programme design and a failure to integrate training components and manipulate training variables results in:

- Generation of high levels of fatigue
- Reduced potential for performance
- A greater risk of injury

Programming the 'Satnav'

When we set out on a car journey, there are several pieces of crucial information that we need in order to ensure we arrive at our destination:

1. Where do we want to go?
2. Where are we starting from?
3. How would we like to get there?
4. The road is closed – now what?

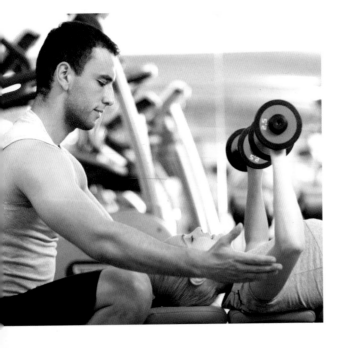

STEP #1: WHERE DO WE WANT TO GO?

The first step is to actually decide on the finishing point (goal). Ask anyone involved in performance sport and they will confirm that they always start with the end in mind and then work backwards. We love to 'reverse engineer' in sport. British Cycling are probably one of the best at this. They figure out what medals they want to win at the next Olympics and then work backwards on their plan. The more detail we can provide about where we want to go, the more chance we have of arriving at the correct location at the right time.

This part of the planning process is all about setting goals (outcome, performance, process) and then making them SMART.

If you have a goal, you have a training purpose.

Goals always determine methods, establish your outcome then work back from there to create something that is deliverable in the time you have available.
Darren Roberts High Performance Manager, Harris and Ross Healthcare

What is your training purpose? Where do you want to go? The first step of the programme design process is to actually decide on the finishing point, developing an understanding of

◁ If you have a goal, you have a training purpose

the 'destination' and figuring out how quickly you want to get there. If you're a regular at the gym, in the pool or at the fitness class, I guarantee you'll have a goal, a training purpose – you just may not realise it! It's unlikely that you are training just for the sake of it and while there may be a few people who simply love to train, I think we can agree that they're in the minority. The chances are that you started to think about physical preparation, getting fit or working out, around the time you set yourself a goal. It could have been to play five-a-side football once a week with your mates, run a marathon, or fit into the suit that's been hanging in your wardrobe for the last 3 years. These are goals and I bet if I dug deep enough I could find a goal or training purpose for everyone reading this book. The problem is that most of you will have done a decidedly average job of setting your training goal, so this is probably a good point to take a look at how to establish effective training goals before we move on to look at the needs analysis. A ton of information exists on goal setting so I'll try to keep it brief! There are three different types of goals that you can set yourself and they tend to be interlinked:

1. Outcome
2. Performance
3. Process

Outcome Goals

This type of goal is typically linked to a desired end result, e.g. I want to fit into my skinny jeans or I want to win the cup final with my Sunday league team. This type of goal paints a picture and can be great for motivation, but there's

a big problem if the only goal you set is an outcome goal.

An outcome goal is not always under your control and can often be affected by how others perform. What if you set an outcome goal of finishing a half-marathon in the top 50 for your age group but on the day you finish 51st, despite running your perfect race. You've failed! You've missed your goal. Outcome goals are of limited use if they are not related to process and performance goals.

'Actions create the habit. Goals define the actions. Your outcomes define the goals. Keep the three areas separate in your mind. People with too much focus on the end outcome get frustrated and make bad choices that prevent habits being formed. Planning starts big to small. Habit building starts small to big.'

Richard Nugent M.D., TwentyOne Leadership and Success In Football

Performance Goals

Performance goals specify a standard to be achieved. A performance goal is under your control. Performance goals are about setting yourself targets that are unaffected by the performance of others. Using the example of a top 50 half-marathon finish, let's say you've figured out that in order to do that you need to run a 1 hour 45 minute half-marathon. To do that, you need to run at an even 8:01 minutes per mile pace. If you run an even race at that pace you achieve your 'performance goal', but maybe finish 51st and miss your 'outcome goal'. This is fine; you've done everything you could to achieve your outcome goal but on the day were beaten by someone faster. You've still run the perfect race and hit your performance goal. Performance goals are really important to have and are often overlooked.

Process Goals

Process goals take the outcome goal and performance goal and add a final layer of strategy. Sticking with our half-marathon example, if you know you need to run at an 8:01 minute per mile pace to achieve your performance goal of 1 hour 45 minutes to give yourself a chance of achieving your 'outcome goal' of a top 50 finish, then you need to have a strategy – a plan. Process goals could be:

- Improve lower limb strength levels by following a structured training programme for 8 weeks
- Complete three strength training sessions each week
- Improve running technique

A crucial part of the planning process is to establish a goal, making sure you have thought about not only the outcome, but the performance and process goals too. Once you have your goal in place, you need to make sure that each goal is SMART.

- **Specific –** 'I want to get in shape' is not very specific, in fact it's about as 'woolly' as you can get, but this is the opening statement I heard time and time again from prospective clients when I ran a private training facility. What sort of shape do you want to be? Round, oblong, skinny, hench? The devil really is in the detail so get specific. 'I want

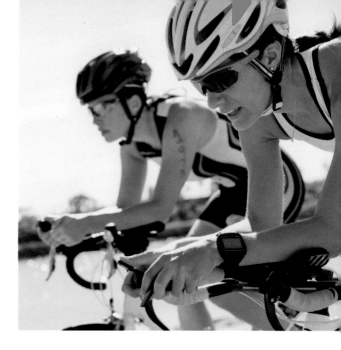

to be able to jog for 10 minutes, three times a week.'
- **Measurable –** One of the most important lessons you can take from athletes is that they measure progress throughout their career. Ideally, you want an objective measure of your progress. It could be that little black dress hanging in the wardrobe because the zip won't do up, or a 'personal best' time that you're aiming for over a 10km course. The moment the zip on that black dress slides up easily or you break your PB by 10 seconds is the moment you know you've achieved your goal. It's measurable.
- **Agreed –** When I work with athletes and teams, we have to have agreement on the overall goal, otherwise there are going to be problems ahead. Anyone who is involved in your success needs to be signed up. I've worked with numerous recreational triathletes, many of whom I've helped to prepare for the ultimate challenge of an Ironman. Now, an Ironman is a challenging

event, not least for the fact that you are taking three tough disciplines: swimming 2.4 miles, cycling 112 miles and running 26.2 miles (that's a marathon to you and me!) and putting them all together in one event. The event itself is gruelling so you can only imagine how tough the training is. Many of the recreational triathletes I trained were successful business people juggling the demands of work, home life and training. Not all of them had agreement from the people who played a crucial role in their success (colleagues, family, friends, etc). Disappearing out of the house on a Sunday morning for what will essentially be the whole day to put some miles in on the bike can wear a little thin with family members and could ultimately scupper your chances of success, unless they are fully on board with what you are trying to achieve. Get agreement from the outset.

- **Realistic –** 'I want to be able to run the Great North Run, Nick' is not an unusual request, but as a coach I have to figure out if this is a realistic goal. Goals have to be challenging, they have to make you stretch for something that is just out of reach, but you can't shoot for the stars straight away (don't pick your first fight with a Ninja!). I make my decision based on a needs analysis and while I believe pretty much everything is achievable, we have to be realistic about how and what we are going to do.

- **Timed –** Probably the most powerful element of goal setting is to fix a target date. Nothing concentrates the mind like a deadline! I've lost track of how many times I've entered an event only to get the 'fear' as

soon as I've received the confirmation email from the organisers that my entry has been accepted. Once you've entered, you have your time frame – better get training! Time frames dictate how we approach the task. If time is tight, you may need to dedicate more time to your training or adjust other elements of your goal.

 Prioritise your goals

You often find that you'll be working on several goals so you'll need to prioritise them. Often it's related to the time frames you're working towards, so think about short- and long-term goals and how each impacts on the other. Write it down – this is a simple yet powerful tool. Once you've established your goal, write it down and you'll be amazed because something magical happens when you put pen to paper! Stick up your written goal somewhere where you'll see it every day and – even better – tell someone about your goal. There's nothing like a friend asking you how you're getting on with your training to ensure you stay on track!

STEP #2: WHERE ARE WE STARTING FROM?

The second step of setting up the satnav is to establish the starting point. In order to know where the journey starts, the satnav needs to establish a strong satellite signal that will provide enough information to tell the satnav where the journey begins. The first step of a training process is to complete a detailed initial needs analysis.

Needs Analysis

Where are we? Once you've figured out your training purpose (goal), you should set about working through a needs analysis. This is the next step you need to take before you start thinking about writing a training programme. You may think this is a waste of time and want to skip this section to start working on your training programme, but if it's good enough for athletes and sports teams then it's good enough for you.

A needs analysis is simply the process of pulling together all the information you require to provide you with a clear understanding of where you are at this precise moment in time. It's a bit like taking a photo – you need to capture the moment and then figure out how to move forwards.

The entire process of programme design needs to be individualised. A thorough needs analysis is a major step in determining exactly what exercises you will need to perform at each stage of your long-term programme and the information you gather ensures that you optimise the programme design process. Let's take a look at what I believe are the key areas you need to think about and the questions covering the areas of lifestyle, fitness, health and performance that you should ask yourself when completing your needs analysis.

Lifestyle

The success or failure of your training programme will be heavily influenced by your lifestyle but this is often an area that is overlooked. Your day-to-day living will shape how much training you can complete, when you can take part in fitness sessions, how long those sessions will last and how quickly you will recover from training. It's worth taking some time and figuring out some basic lifestyle information.

- **Work/school commitments –** How much time each week do you spend at work/school/college? Knowing when you can actually train will influence how you put your programme together.
- **Travel time –** How much time do you spend travelling to and from work, school, etc? This is often overlooked but I learned my lesson some years ago when I worked with the England Netball team. We figured out that our players were spending a considerable amount of time travelling to and from training, which had a negative impact on their recovery and regeneration and training quality. I now take this area into consideration with every athlete I work with.
- **Demanding job –** Is your job mentally or physically demanding? If you're in your final year at university, the mental demands of sitting your final exams and writing a dissertation could be huge and you need to think about the impact this may have on training. Equally, if you have a physically demanding job you'll more than likely carry residual fatigue from work into every training session.
- **Sedentary work –** Do you have a sedentary job, slumped in front of a computer all day? If so, there's a high chance that you'll have adopted some postural patterns that may

not be conducive to your training or sport and that will need to be addressed in the training programme. I like to know how long my clients spend sitting at a desk and how their workstation is set up.

- **Sleep –** What are your sleeping habits (time to bed, hours in bed, quality of sleep)? Sleep is one of the most important forms of rest and provides time for you to adapt to the physical and mental demands of training. We've seen in earlier sections of the book the importance of recovery and regeneration and the link between sleep and training quality and performance outcomes. If your training adaptations have hit a plateau, it could simply be down to the fact that your sleeping habits are poor and you're not giving your body a chance to recover and adapt. Studies have shown that as little as 30–36 hours of sleep deprivation can result in a loss of performance (physical, mental). Those hours don't all have to occur at the same time, they can be accumulated over a period of time. Cutting back on your sleep over the course of a week could push you into sleep debt.

- **Nutrition** – Training performance is inextricably linked to nutritional habits and optimal performance and training adaptations can only occur when the body is fuelled appropriately. Have you ever sat down and thought about your eating habits?

  - How many meals do you eat per day?
  - What are the timings of the meals?
  - Do you take any supplements?
  - Do you like to cook?
  - What's your favourite type of food?

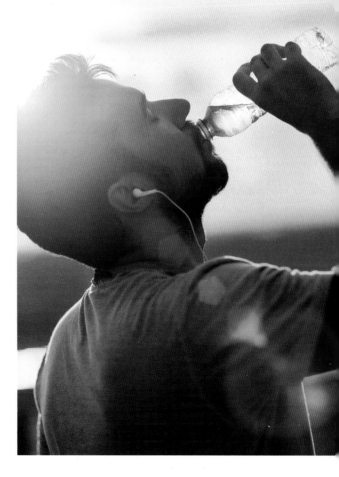

Taking the time to review your nutritional habits is a really useful exercise and some simple changes could boost your performances. Are you getting the basics right?

- Eat regularly
- Go easy on sugars and processed food
- Eat fruit and vegetables
- Drink plenty of water (2.5 litres per day)

Fitness

Fitness relates to your physical preparation and your ability to perform particular tasks. People often embark on a training programme without first considering their current fitness status. One of my favourite sayings is 'The older I get, the better I was', and when embarking on a new training programme we sometimes forget that it's been a while since we actually trained! Take some time to consider the following points:

- Are you currently training? If so, how often and for how long?
- Where are you currently training? Do you need access to specialised training facilities or can you just head out on the streets for a run?
- When was the last time you trained? Remember the 'use/disuse' cornerstone. This is particularly important when you're returning to fitness. Make sure you take time to build your training back up. Most programmes fail in the first week because people train so hard that they end up with either an injury or so much muscle soreness it puts them off exercise for another decade!
- What type of training do you like and dislike? When I work with professional athletes I tell them that sometimes they are going to have to do things they don't particularly enjoy. For them, it's a job, and just like any job we have tasks that need to be done and we don't always relish the idea of doing them. This may hold true for you, too, but it's worth noting that if you hate working out in a gym then you're unlikely to stick to your programme if it means every session is spent there. Identify what you like to do to keep fit and then select activities that are going to give you the best chance of success.

Health

Health covers your medical and health status. Understanding your medical history is important prior to embarking on a programme of physical preparation. If you are not healthy, you can't train to the best of your ability, and progress will be limited. Taking the time to review your current health status is a really useful exercise and some simple changes to your lifestyle could boost your health and well-being. Take some time to consider the following questions:

- Have you had any major surgeries?
- Are you currently taking any medications?
- Are you currently suffering from any ongoing medical conditions?
- Do you suffer from regular headaches?
- Do you suffer from unusual levels of fatigue or have a general lack of energy?

 Injury History

If you've had an injury you will know that it ruins motivation and can lead to significant performance decrements. Understanding your 'injury profile' could provide clues about your current training programme and where it may need to be improved or developed.
- Have you broken any bones?
- Do you suffer from back pain?
- Make a list of your recent injuries (within last 2 years)
- Make a list of your major injuries (including ones from more than 2 years ago)

Performance

What is it that you want to be able to do? If you've done a thorough job of establishing your training purpose (goal), this section should be pretty simple to complete. Much of what you need to consider will be drawn out from the performance and process goals. Even if you're not training to take part in a sporting event, you should still consider your 'training purpose'. If you want simply to be fit enough to play with your grandchildren when they come to visit, you can still work through this section.

- What are the demands of the sport, event or activity that you will be taking part in or are training for?
- What are your strengths and weaknesses? If you struggle to answer this question, consider how you can be beaten. What's your 'Kryptonite'?
- Does the team you play for have a particular 'playing philosophy' or style? For example, if you're taking part in an adventure race, does your team want to complete the course as quickly as possible or do you just want to survive and make it to the end for a well-earned pint?
- When are the major competitions that you are preparing for? When does your season start and finish?

Before selecting your tools, make sure you understand the performance question. Always match the tool to the question and never the other way around.

Mark Jarvis MSc. Director of Performance Solutions, English Institute of Sport

STEP #3 HOW WOULD WE LIKE TO GET THERE?

The third step is to select the route. The satnav usually provides you with some options: do you want to take the quickest route, would you like to take the most direct route, would you like to avoid certain locations and do you want to avoid paying any road tolls! The programme you develop will be influenced by the first two steps (goal setting and needs analysis). Armed with this information, you can now develop the structured programme (route) to take you from point A to point B.

There's a difference between a workout, and a programme. A programme is more than a series of workouts. A programme has direction, structure, development and purpose.

Alwyn Cosgrove. Owner, Results Fitness

Periodisation

Which way will we go? Once you've established your training goal (remember, everyone should be training with a purpose) and completed a needs analysis, you'll have to sit down and think about the training programme that is going to help take you from where you are now to your final destination. The programme you develop will be influenced by the first two steps and should help you progress towards your goal(s).

Periodisation and programme design is all about the development of a structured programme that divides your training into manageable phases. The periodised training programme is the 'blueprint' that you'll work from. Each training phase should have sufficient variation in the training stimuli (you'll learn how to manipulate a range of training variables later in this section) and incorporate planned rest periods to improve recovery and restoration and increase the potential for achieving specific performance goals.

> There's a huge difference between writing and completing a training session and a training programme.

Training plans can be extremely complicated but I believe they should be kept as simple as possible and flexible enough to be adapted and modified as training progresses. When you sit down to write a plan to help you achieve a goal, you need some structure and your programmes should be designed with both short- and long-term objectives in mind. Thankfully, some clever coaches based in Eastern Europe set about creating a logical system of training back in the 1950s, and their pioneering work has gone on to inform programme design ever since. At the core of their work is the fact that a training plan can be broken down into logical sequential components. I liken the components of a periodised plan to Russian dolls (a set of wooden dolls of decreasing size placed one inside the other).

Russian dolls

The Russian doll is a design classic that shows the relationship of an 'object within a similar object'. The building blocks of a periodised programme are very similar in nature: each step is related to the other and, as the programme is developed, the layers of information and complexity also increase.

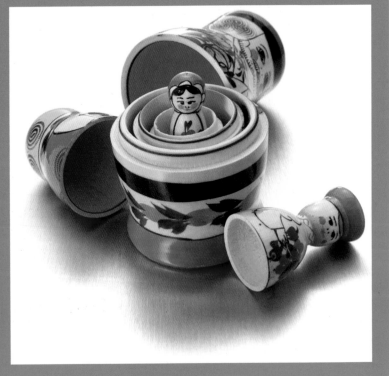

MACROCYCLE | THE BIG PICTURE

Macrocycle: the big picture

- **Macrocycle – the complete plan –** This is the 'Mummy' Russian doll – the largest one, which conceals all the other layers. The macrocycle is 'THE BIG PICTURE' and reflects one complete cycle. Typically, it lasts a year; however, I believe it can be shorter or longer and should essentially be linked to your ultimate training goal. If you have 6 months to get ready for a marathon, the macrocycle can be 6 months.

  When you are putting together your macrocycle, you need to consider all the 'immovable objects'. Make a note of all the things that can't be changed, e.g. competition dates, holidays and school exam periods. Understanding where your 'immovable objects' are placed will help you when you take your plan to the next level of detail.

  You can break the macrocycle down further into three distinct phases – preparation, competition and transition – and if you want to get really technical you can break each of these phases down further, into general preparation and specific preparation, early competition, mid competition and late competition. (Now you know why I've gone for the Russian doll metaphor!).

- **Mesocycle – several continuous weeks of training –** A mesocycle is a number of continuous weeks (typically 4–6) within the macrocycle where the training programme emphasises the same type of physical adaptations. It can be thought of as the 'monthly plan'. If your needs analysis has identified that you need to improve your relative strength, you may spend a mesocycle during the specific preparation phase of the macrocycle focusing your training on developing this physical quality. If your training priority is to improve your flexibility and mobility so that you can perform your strength training with better technique, this would be emphasised in a mesocycle. The physical adaptations that you gain during this mesocycle should have a positive impact on the physical quality

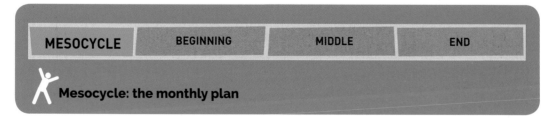

MESOCYCLE | BEGINNING | MIDDLE | END

Mesocycle: the monthly plan

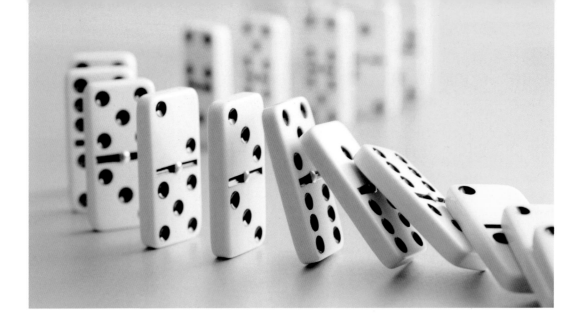

you are working on in the next mesocycle. Think of it like a row of dominoes (I'm sure you've watched world record domino runs, each domino falling and knocking the next one to create a cascade of dominoes). This is what you are trying to achieve with your mesocycle. The positive physical adaptations gained in one mesocycle should have a 'knock-on' effect, leading to positive gains in the next mesocycle.

- **Microcycle – typically a 7-day period but can range from 5–10 days –** A microcycle often lasts for seven days and is a training week within the mesocycle. This will be your 'weekly plan', providing you with details of specific training sessions that need to be completed that week.

STEP #4 THE ROAD IS CLOSED – NOW WHAT?

Once you've started out on the journey, you need to be prepared to make changes based on traffic updates. An initial needs analysis has limited use if you fail to follow up with regular updates. These will provide you with important pieces of information relating to your progress.

> Programme design is a 'process' and you must be prepared to make changes to the route if necessary.

Training programmes must balance the need for continuity while taking into account the

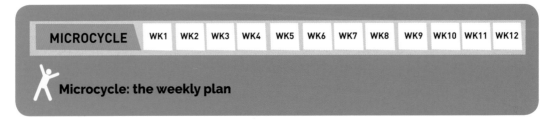

| MICROCYCLE | WK1 | WK2 | WK3 | WK4 | WK5 | WK6 | WK7 | WK8 | WK9 | WK10 | WK11 | WK12 |

Microcycle: the weekly plan

importance of variation. Ongoing monitoring of your progress will allow you to track the rate of change and provide clues as to when it's time to freshen up the programme. You may adapt to a training session in as little as three to six exposures to the same stimulus. Once you've adapted to the training stimulus, make a change. As a general rule, look to manipulate the training variables within the programme every 4–6 weeks to ensure you continue to progress and improve. Take into account your training history; if you're a novice, you may not cope too well with lots of significant changes to your training programme, so if the programme still works, stick with it.

> When I first started out as a strength and conditioning coach, I would write completely new training programmes for my athletes every 4–6 weeks. When I say completely new, I mean it – everything changed! I realised after about 3 months that this was not the best approach (if for no other reason than I ran out of exercises!). As I've developed as a coach, I've recognised that small changes to one or two training variables can have a significant impact on the outcomes of a training programme. It's all about evolution – not revolution!

Training Variables

In Chapter 3 you learned about the cornerstones of developing an integrated performance conditioning programme. These cornerstones will underpin your understanding of how to manipulate training variables, and how they can be managed to enhance performance. A huge amount has been written on programme design and it's often very confusing. Here, I'll provide you with an overview of the key training variables that can be manipulated to bring about changes in your programme and performance.

VOLUME

Training volume is possibly the single most important variable. It needs to be manipulated with care in order to avoid overreaching and overtraining. In my experience, most fitness enthusiasts adopt a 'results by volume' approach to their training. This is a common mistake, based on the belief that if you simply do more work you'll become better.

Training volume is the total amount of training performed during a specific period of time and can be measured per session, day, week, month or year. If we look at some typical exercises as an example, we can quickly work out what the training volume will be.

- Back Squat: 4 sets of 8 repetitions with 50kg would have a training volume of 1600kg (4 x 8 x 50 = 1600)
- Interval Running: 4 sets of 5 repetitions covering 100m each repetition would have a training volume of 2000 meters (1.2 miles) (4 x 5 x 100 = 2000)

We know from earlier chapters that one of the key components of an IPC is training with intent (intensity). One of the most important training concepts to keep at the forefront of your mind is that volume is inversely related to intensity. What does that mean? In its simplest terms, if you have high training volumes then training intensity will have to be low, and vice versa. You can't deliver large volumes of high-intensity training for extended periods of time (well, you could try but it will only end up with one outcome – overtraining). It's worth remembering that physical preparation is cumulative (remember the analogy of putting £10 in the bank every day) – it's not how much training is completed in one training session that is important, it's how much training is completed during a training week, month and year. Keeping tabs on your training volume will allow you to programme weeks that allow for recovery as well as weeks that push you to your limits. If you don't track training volume, how will you know which is which?

INTENSITY

The overall aim of a training programme is to develop your ability to train at a higher level, at increasingly higher intensities

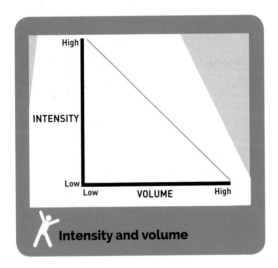

Intensity and volume

(degree of effort, expressed as a percentage of maximum capacity). Training intensity is another important training variable that can be manipulated to bring about overload and two factors have a significant impact when programming training intensity:

1. **Volume** – There is an inverse relationship between volume and intensity. I've mentioned that already!
2. **Recovery** – Intensity is recovery-dependent. If you're not fully recovered, training intensity is going to be compromised.

So how hard should you train? A common response may be, 'Go hard or go home!' I like to think we are a little bit more sophisticated than that, and one of the simplest methods for gauging training intensity was developed by Australian strength and conditioning expert Ian King. I've used this simple scale for more than a decade and it's always worked really well for me:

■ Level One: No Fatigue – easy
■ Level Two: Medium Fatigue – could have completed at least one more repetition
■ Level Three: High Fatigue – could not have completed another repetition
■ Level Four: Failure – failed during a repetition
■ Level Five: Beyond Failure – used 'forced' reps to complete the set

I would suggest that for most of you reading this book, you will never need to hit level five – to my mind, once you've failed during a repetition, your set is completed.

Modern technology allows us to use more sophisticated measures of training intensity but this simple method works a treat.

> When programming training volume and intensity, you must always remember the 'individual differences' cornerstone and consider other factors that can impact on training intensity (training age, chronological age, gender, genetic blueprint).

TRAINING AVAILABILITY

How often can you actually train? This is often overlooked when developing a training programme, but it can have a massive impact on the overall success of your training. When I ask clients how often they can train, I usually get a standard answer: 'I could train three times a week for about an hour.' What they really mean is that by the time they've done everything else in their day-to-day life they'll realistically be able to commit to two sessions of 30–45 minutes. This isn't a problem; you just need to be honest, because training availability will change the overall complexion of your training programme and also dictate how quickly you will be able to achieve your goals. Your availability to train, or density (total number of sessions or units completed within a time frame, e.g. four sessions per week), is often overlooked during programme design but is an important element to consider and can have a huge impact on rate of progression.

> Take some time to figure out how often you'll be able to train each week. Complete the weekly planner below to get a feel for your training availability.

There are two elements that need to be considered when you sit down to figure out your training availability.

1. Frequency

Training frequency refers to the number of training sessions completed during a period

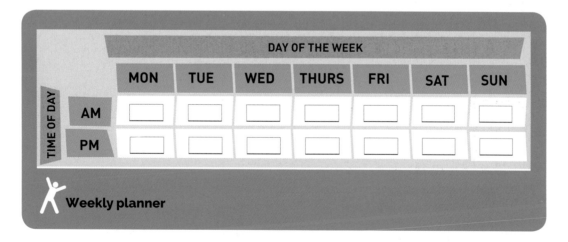

		MON	TUE	WED	THURS	FRI	SAT	SUN
TIME OF DAY	**AM**							
	PM							

Weekly planner

of time (week, month etc). You need to figure out how many days you can train in a week. Research indicates that optimal improvements in training occur when you are able to train at least three times per week, although research also indicates that if training intensity is kept at an appropriate level, fitness can be maintained with just one training session a week. Determining the frequency of workouts per week has a huge impact on how quickly you can achieve performance outcomes and the overall success of your programme.

An inverse relationship exists between training frequency and both training intensity and training volume. What this basically means is that if you plan on completing either really high-intensity training sessions or high volumes of work in a training session, you are not going to be able to cope with performing multiple training sessions (high frequency). The simple fact of the matter is that your body needs time to recover and your ability to put together multiple training efforts during a week will be dependent on residual fatigue and the ability to recover from training.

When programming training frequency, you must always remember the 'individual differences' cornerstone and consider other factors that can impact on training intensity (training age, chronological age, gender, genetic blueprint, size of muscle and number of muscle groups being trained. We are all different, and how we cope with the demands of a training programme will differ from person to person!

 How often can you train each week?

- 1–2 days a week – This level of training will suit you if you have a busy lifestyle with other commitments. You have to accept that your rate of progress will be limited and your training will have to be more general in nature.
- 3–4 days a week – If you are looking to optimise training adaptations, you will benefit from training more regularly. Recovery must be taken into consideration to make sure you actually get the adaptations you are chasing.

It's important to consider when you are able to complete your training sessions because this will also impact on your training progression. What if your working week means you can only train at the weekends? While it is possible to complete back-to-back workouts during a training week, the fatigue of workout A may influence the training effect of workout B.

2. Duration

Training duration in its simplest form is the total training time (duration in minutes or hours from start to end of the training session, e.g. 90 minutes). The duration of a training session is a function of reps, sets, number of exercises and recovery. It's simple mathematics and below are a couple of examples of how each element is related and creates a total training time.

Exercise	Sets	Reps	Tempo	Rest	Time to complete exercise
Squat	4	8	1 0 1	120 secs	9 minutes
Stiff Leg Deadlift	4	8	1 0 1	120 secs	9 minutes
Push-up	4	10	2 1 2	60 secs	7 minutes
Inverse Pull	4	8	1 0 1	60 secs	5 minutes
Chin-up	3	5	1 0 1	60 secs	4 minutes
TOTAL TRAINING TIME – 34 MINUTES					

This session would take 34 minutes to complete, and that doesn't take into account time spent warming up and cooling down, chatting to your friends and going over your specified rest time!

 Table 9.1

You can do the same for an interval session.

Training Session	Sets	Reps	Work	Rest	Time to complete exercise
Broken 100s	4	5	30	30 secs	20 minutes
Recovery between sets – 3 minutes	9 minutes				
TOTAL TRAINING TIME – 29 MINUTES					

This session would take 29 minutes to complete, and that doesn't take into account time spent warming up and cooling down, chatting to your friends and going over your specified rest time!

 Table 9.2

With an understanding of the interrelationship of each variable and its impact on session duration, you can now start to see how long your planned sessions are going to take and what impact that may have on your training availability during the rest of the week.

Session duration will ultimately have an impact on 'available energy'; once the 'tanks' are empty you can't continue, so you'll need to either stop and recover or refuel appropriately throughout the training session. It's worth bearing in mind that training sessions that exceed 60–90 minutes are associated with catabolic processes that disturb hormonal and immune system responses. These hormonal responses can have a negative impact on training and health, which is why I like to keep training sessions short and sweet. Get in – get your session done – go home!

MODALITY

Training modality refers to the type of training that you will be completing. When considering training modality, take time to reflect on the 'specificity' cornerstone: the body will adapt specifically to the overload stimulus placed upon it. The type of training that you complete should be specific and relate closely to your training goals. Training type can be viewed at two levels:

- Level 1 – General: strength, speed, metabolic, flexibility
- Level 2 – Specific: sub-components of the general quality, e.g. speed (change of direction or linear acceleration)

If my training goal is to complete an adventure race that requires a lot of off-road running, including a significant amount of hill climbing, I need to consider carefully the training modality. Sure, I need to work on my metabolic conditioning but I have to consider more specifically the sub-components of metabolic conditioning that ought to be addressed. At

some point in my training plan, I will need to include some efforts that challenge the specific energy systems that will be called upon during a hill climb.

REPETITION

The number of repetitions performed is arguably the single most important micro variable that we can manipulate.

A repetition is one complete movement of a particular exercise and is simply a method of counting the number of movements performed without rest. For example, if you perform a push-up 10 times in a row without stopping, you have completed 10 reps. All micro variables are interdependent and will have an impact on other variables. If you decide to use a repetition range of 15, this will immediately have an influence on the number of sets you can perform (there is an inverse relationship between repetitions and sets) and the choice of exercise.

Training within a specific range of repetitions will produce specific adaptations (see p. 121). One of the most important training concepts to consider is the 'repetition continuum' and the inverse relationship between reps and sets.

Exercise	Sets	Reps	Tempo	Rest
A	3	8	1 0 1	60 seconds
B	3	8	1 0 1	60 seconds
C	3	8	1 0 1	60 seconds
D	3	8	1 0 1	60 seconds

 Table 9.3

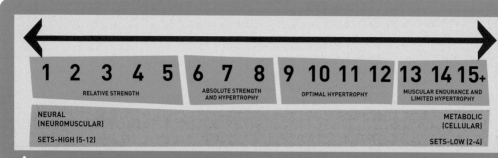

1	**2**	**3**	**4**	**5**	**6**	**7**	**8**	**9**	**10**	**11**	**12**	**13**	**14**	**15+**
	RELATIVE STRENGTH				ABSOLUTE STRENGTH AND HYPERTROPHY			OPTIMAL HYPERTROPHY				MUSCULAR ENDURANCE AND LIMITED HYPERTROPHY		

NEURAL
(NEUROMUSCULAR)

METABOLIC
(CELLULAR)

SETS-HIGH (5-12)

SETS-LOW (2-4)

The Repetition Continuum

Adjusting the repetitions for a given exercise can be a very powerful stimulus that will boost your training adaptations. You'll often see coaches chopping and changing exercises every 4 weeks in an attempt to bring about a training adaptation. My advice: don't look to change exercises radically (the body adapts slowly to changes in exercise). Stick to the same exercise but switch up your repetition range for faster results.

When programming repetitions, you must always remember the 'individual differences' cornerstone and consider other factors that can impact on training intensity (training age, chronological age, gender, genetic blueprint).

SETS

A set is a group of consecutive repetitions performed with rests between sets. For example, if you complete 10 reps on bench press, this is your first set. If you then complete another 10 repetitions on bench press, you have completed your second set and so on.

> **A set is a group of consecutive repetitions.**

There is an inverse relationship between sets and reps. Remember, repetitions control pretty much everything else when it comes

Exercise	Sets	Reps	Tempo	Rest
A	**3**	8	1 0 1	60 seconds
B	**3**	8	1 0 1	60 seconds
C	**3**	8	1 0 1	60 seconds
D	**3**	8	1 0 1	60 seconds

Table 9.4

to programme design and the relationship between these two variables will ultimately impact on training intensity. The number of sets per exercise is also inversely related to the number of exercises. You can't programme a large number of exercises and a high number of sets. Well, you can, but it will be a long session and that goes against one of our key points in the training blueprint – efficiency. Why would you want to spend any more time than was absolutely necessary working out in the gym! Conditioning-based activities requiring a greater metabolic stimulus typically have more sets, while power-based activities requiring a greater neural stimulus have fewer sets.

> When programming the number of sets, do no more than absolutely necessary – if in doubt, do less! There has been a growing trend to follow training programmes that encourage high training volumes, 'doing work' under the misguided notion that the more work completed, the better the training session. Forget it. I would much rather my athletes train 'harder' while performing fewer sets.

Set configuration can have an impact on programme design and performance outcomes and once again you'll see coaches prescribing some elaborate set configurations in an attempt to optimise performance. In my humble opinion, the majority of you will achieve great gains by using one of these simple configurations.

Traditional

There's nothing wrong with sticking to the basics and building your programme around a traditional set configuration. In the traditional model, each repetition is performed with no rest between the repetitions in each set. At the end of the set, you take a rest and then perform the next set for the same exercise. Your programme will look like Table 9.5.

Superset

The superset is a great approach when you want to ensure your training efficiency is maintained (remember – no medals for being in the gym the longest!) and you want to optimise the amount of work that can be completed within a training session. If you opt to use the superset approach, you will combine two or more exercises (typically upper and

Exercise	Sets	Reps	Tempo	Rest
A	3	8	1 0 1	60 seconds
B	3	8	1 0 1	60 seconds
C	3	8	1 0 1	60 seconds
D	3	8	1 0 1	60 seconds

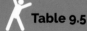 Table 9.5

lower body or different body parts, e.g. quadriceps and hamstrings), but this time you complete all the reps for the first set of the first exercise then, without resting, move straight to the next exercise and complete all the reps for the first set of the second exercise.

Strength and conditioning purists will probably get a little upset by what I'm about to suggest. Supersets traditionally don't have rest periods between each exercise; however, I programme a short rest period (15–30 seconds) between each exercise. Once all the sets and reps of the superset have been completed. I then programme in a longer rest period – 60–120 seconds – before moving on to complete the next superset. Why? Well, it's based on reality. Chances are you are training in a gym with other members and you can't have all your work stations set up for your exclusive use, so it's highly likely that there's going to be some rest between sets and I like to make sure it's programmed and taken into account. If you use a superset structure, your programme will look like Table 9.6.

Using the example below, you would complete the exercises as follows:

- Complete first set of 1A
- Recover (30 seconds)
- Move to 1B and complete the first set (recover 30 seconds)
- Repeat until all sets have been completed for exercises 1A and 1B

Contrast

A contrast set is simply the combination of a resistance exercise (heavy load) with a matched explosive exercise (lighter load). This form of training is great for a number of reasons but at its most basic level it's a time-efficient method of training and allows you to work on two different but complementary components of strength. Your training programme will look like Table 9.7.

You'll notice that the rest period between the first and second exercise is minimal – just 30 seconds – but the rest after the second exercise (before completing the next set of the first exercise) is longer – 120 seconds.

Exercise	Sets	Reps	Tempo	Rest
1A	3	8	1 0 1	**30 seconds**
1B	3	8	1 0 1	**30 seconds**
2A	3	8	1 0 1	**30 seconds**
2B	3	8	1 0 1	**30 seconds**

 Table 9.6

Exercise	Sets	Reps	Tempo	Rest
1A	3	8	1 0 1	30 seconds
1B	3	8	1 0 1	120 seconds
2A	3	8	1 0 1	30 seconds
2B	3	8	1 0 1	120 seconds

Table 9.7

Load

Training load (the amount of weight lifted) should also be programmed with 'specificity' in mind. Load will dictate the speed of movement (tempo) and force production, both of which impact on specific performance outcomes. So how much should you lift? It all depends on what your training goals are. If you want to get strong, you will lift heavier loads than you would if you were training for hypertrophy. Typically, there is an inverse relationship between load and repetitions (high load – low reps, low load – high reps). However, it's worth remembering the 'individual differences' cornerstone and considering other factors that can impact on training load. For example,

I often programme beginners to train with a low load, working in a low repetition range (<5) typically associated with development of relative strength qualities. Clearly, with a light load I'm not chasing improvements in relative strength. What I'm looking for is an opportunity to allow for greater coaching input between sets and to establish technique without fatigue. If I programme high repetitions (>12), technique may break down early on in the set, say after 4 repetitions, and then I'm left coaching 8 repetitions with poor technique. When we are trying to establish technique, it's obvious that the 8 repetitions with poor technique are going to override the learning process taking place during the 4 good repetitions.

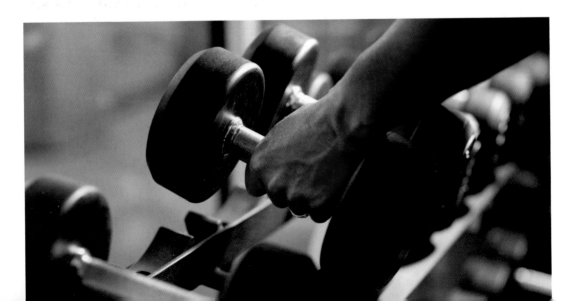

Speed of Movement

Speed of movement should always be programmed with 'specificity' in mind but it is often overlooked or poorly programmed by coaches and athletes and this can create all sorts of problems. Speed of movement, or 'tempo', is an important variable that can be used to achieve specific training outcomes and is an element of programme design that allows you to adjust the duration of the repetition. The speed at which each repetition is performed can be expressed as a percentage of maximum effort (e.g. endurance training – run 20 minutes at 75 per cent) or as a unit of time (e.g. take 2 seconds to lower the bar, 1 second pause at the bottom and 1 second to raise the bar). The strength and conditioning coach Ian King pioneered the concept of tempo for resistance training and provided some simple training guidelines in his book *How To Write Strength Training Programmes*. Putting together a programme with inappropriate tempos can result in a Time Under Tension (TUT) that is detrimental to the overall training goal.

> Time Under Tension (TUT) is a term used to describe the time the muscle is working continuously and is related to speed of movement. Neural adaptations tend to occur <40 seconds (short TUT) and metabolic adaptations tend to occur >40 seconds (long TUT).

Let's say your training goal was to develop functional hypertrophy and you selected a repetition range of 12 to bring about the training adaptations that you are looking for (metabolic). Banging out 12 repetitions with a very quick tempo will see you finishing that exercise in under 40 seconds (we've all witnessed this in the gym – someone slides under the bar and completes their set in the blink of an eye), missing out on the metabolic adaptations that you are chasing. In order to get the most from your 12 repetitions, you would need to make sure that each repetition lasted at least 3–4 seconds.

I don't want to over-complicate things in this book, so the key points you need to consider when producing a strength training programme are:

- Select your repetitions
- Take into account the type of adaptation that training within this repetition range will bring about (neural or metabolic)
- Programme appropriate lifting tempos

When writing a lifting tempo, I've opted for a really simple three-digit method. Other variations exist but in my experience they tend to confuse matters and I've used this approach for many years to good effect. Each digit reflects a part of the lift:

- First digit – first movement
- Second digit – transition or pause
- Third digit – second movement

Let's look at a couple of exercises to give you an example of how it works.

If I programmed a squat with a 2 1 1 tempo, that would mean that I lowered the bar to the bottom of the squat in 2 seconds. I would then pause at the bottom for 1 second before returning to the top of the lift in 1 second. The total TUT for 1 repetition would be 4 seconds.

Exercise	Sets	Reps	Tempo	Rest
Squat	3	5	**2 1 1**	90 seconds

 Table 9.8

If I programmed a chin-up with a 2 2 2 tempo, that would mean that I pulled myself up to the bar in 2 seconds, paused for 2 seconds at the top of the lift and lowered myself back to the starting position in 2 seconds.

Exercise	Sets	Reps	Tempo	Rest
Chin-up	3	5	**2 2 2**	90 seconds

 Table 9.9

If I performed an Olympic lift such as the snatch, I would simply programme 'X', which tells me this is an explosive lift and there's only one way the bar is going to move, and that is as quickly as possible.

Exercise	Sets	Reps	Tempo	Rest
Snatch	4	3	**X**	180 seconds

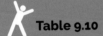 **Table 9.10**

'X' indicates that this should be an explosive movement but remember that the load being used will dictate what that movement actually looks like. If the load is light, the movement will look explosive. If the load is heavy, the bar may move at the speed of a thousand snails, but under these circumstances the 'X' means try to move the bar as quickly as possible: 'an explosive intent'.

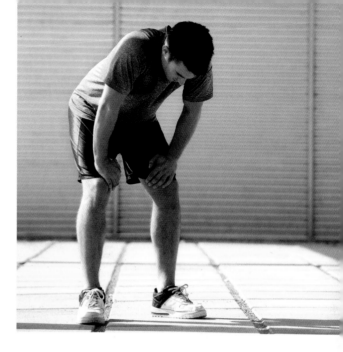

Rarely use 'super slow' tempos (unless rehabilitating from an injury, learning a new technique, or as part of a functional hypertrophy programme). If your training goal is to develop strength and power, the load needs to move with control – but quickly (it's either got to move fast or you need to be trying to move it as fast as possible). Often, the load on the bar will dictate the tempo – just you try sticking to a 'super slow' tempo with a significant amount of weight on the bar!

Recovery

Have you ever taken the time to stop and think about how long you rest between each set? How do you decide when it's time to go again? Hopefully, you'll have given this some consideration but you'll be surprised how many people don't give recovery time the attention it deserves. The rest period is typically the amount of recovery between each set (inter-set recovery is the time taken to recuperate from the last repetition of the set before starting the first repetition of the next set, or exercise.) Depending on your training goals, the rest period between sets can range from 30 seconds to more than 3 minutes. An appropriate rest period can have a massive impact on how well you progress. Your ability to recover between sets is linked to 'available energy'. Once the 'tanks' are empty you can't continue, and to optimise performance, recovery times need to be taken into account. As you can see from the metabolic recovery continuum, the rest

intervals between sets determine the extent to which the energy resources are restored before starting the next set. If you programme 30 seconds' rest between sets, you'll only be 50 per cent recovered. This is fine if you want metabolic adaptations as part of a hypertrophy programme, but it is not so good if you are trying to develop neural adaptations as part of an explosive power development programme.

If you're not convinced that recovery time should be considered carefully, humour me and complete this task. Complete 4 sets of 10 burpees with 30 seconds' rest between each set. In your next training session, complete 4 sets of 10 burpees with 180 seconds' rest between each set. Now tell me that recovery doesn't have an impact on training outcomes.

- **Metabolic – <60 seconds' rest**
- **Neural – >60 seconds' rest**

RECOVERY (%)	50	75	87.5	93.7	97	98.5
TIME (S)	30	60	90	120	150	180

N.B. Neural recovery may take 5-6 times longer than metabolic recovery

 ## Metabolic Recovery Continuum

Typically, an inverse relationship between reps and recovery exists (low reps = high rest) but, as with other training variables, always remember the 'individual differences' cornerstone and consider other factors that can impact on recovery time (training age, chronological age, gender, genetic blueprint, body mass).

Body mass will have an impact on your ability to recover. Experience of working with heavier athletes and private clients (>100kg) would suggest to me that they need longer to recover between sets as the total load (body mass + external load) is greater. Put simply, it's harder work being heavy.

EXERCISE SELECTION

Exercise selection has a significant impact on your training outcomes and it is important to select the most appropriate exercise for optimal performance. Several factors should be considered when selecting exercises but as outlined in Chapter 2 of the book, it is important that you understand the level of functionality of each exercise and how it relates to the performance outcome you want to achieve. Consider every exercise and training session in relation to the outcome.

'*When a weekly programme offers limited opportunity for strength training or conditioning, I tend to go for full body programming.*'

Mark Spivey. B.App.Sci. (Human Movement/Sports Science) ASCC. Director of Fitness and Sport, Radley College (United Kingdom)

Single-joint vs Multi-joint Exercises

Single-joint exercises may be great for targeting hypertrophy within specific muscle groups but it may be more productive and time efficient to use a multi-joint exercise, such as the chin-up, to develop not only the biceps but also other muscles within the upper body.

Bilateral vs Unilateral

Proponents of unilateral training (exercises that work each limb independently of each other) will have you believe that this is the most functional way to train; but if you need to get as strong as possible, you'll be able to shift more weight from using a bilateral exercise such as a squat (both limbs are used together to move the load). It's not really a case of one is better than the other and you'll probably use both approaches at some point in your training. Remember – use the technique that will take you closer to your training goal, not what's currently fashionable.

Stable vs Unstable

It's become trendy to train on unstable surfaces, which is fine if balance and proprioception are important components of your performance outcome. If developing power is the goal of your programme, you will need to make yourself as stable as possible so you can produce as much force as possible. You can't shoot a cannon from a canoe!

Simple vs Complex

Do you pick a simple exercise or a more complicated one? Many strength and conditioning coaches will have you believe that the only way to improve explosive strength is through the use of the Olympic lifts (snatch, clean and jerk). While these are highly effective training techniques, they are also very complex and take time to master. If you have a limited time in which to develop power, I would probably look to use a simple exercise rather than an Olympic lift. Maybe I would programme a contrast set of heavy back squats with box jumps. Why? Well, I can get most people to squat with good technique pretty quickly and jumping up on to a box is another relatively simple technique to teach. If I combine the two techniques, I'm pretty confident I'm going to get decent gains in power. If I decide to work using the snatch, that's going to take time to

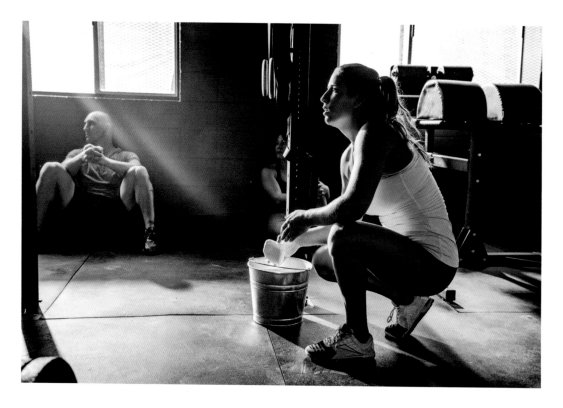

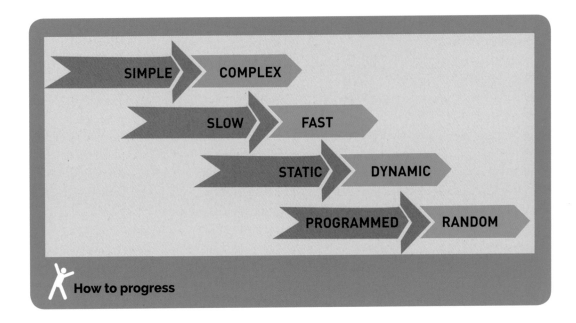

SIMPLE ▶ COMPLEX

SLOW ▶ FAST

STATIC ▶ DYNAMIC

PROGRAMMED ▶ RANDOM

How to progress

perfect and when time is tight it's not going to be my exercise of choice.

In Chapter 3 I highlighted the importance of training the body taking into account how the musculoskeletal system actually functions. Multi-joint exercises using fundamental compound movement patterns are the bedrock of an integrated performance conditioning programme. When selecting exercises, they can be broadly grouped as follows:

■ Knee dominant (e.g. squats, split squats, step-ups)
■ Hip dominant (e.g. deadlift, stiff leg deadlift, supine hip extensions)
■ Vertical push (e.g. shoulder press)
■ Horizontal push (e.g. bench press, push-up, dips)
■ Vertical pull (e.g. chin-up, pull-up)
■ Horizontal pull (e.g. bent over row, inverse pulls)

■ Core rotation (e.g. wood chop, barbell twists, Russian twists)
■ Core stabilisation (e.g. bridge, side hold, plank, roll outs)

EXERCISE SEQUENCE

In what order should you complete your exercises? Several factors must be considered when determining the optimal exercise sequence and these are the two elements that I take into account to figure out the exercise sequence when I'm writing training programmes:

■ **Priority** – This is a pretty good place to start when you are trying to figure out which exercise to complete first. As you progress through the training session, you are going to carry residual fatigue from one exercise to the next. There's little point waiting until the end of the session to complete the most important exercise. If it's important (your training priority), train it first!

- **Complexity** – I generally like to programme the more complex exercises towards the beginning of the training session (with the exception of lower-level movement quality exercises that may be used at the start to 'prime' the next exercise). I think there are physiological benefits (less residual fatigue) as well as psychological benefits (you have to 'switch on' and concentrate straight away, which improves the overall quality of the training session). Linked to the complexity of an exercise is the speed of execution. Again, I generally programme movements that require quick movements towards the start of a training session.

To achieve consistent results from your training, you must be able to develop integrated training programmes. A well-designed training programme should systematically organise your training to provide progression over a period of time, allowing you to achieve your performance outcome. Use the programme design checklist to guide your programme design.

'To be successful with your training, planning is not optional!'

Duncan French PhD, ASCC, CSCS, ASCA-L2. Technical Lead for Strength & Conditioning, English Institute of Sport

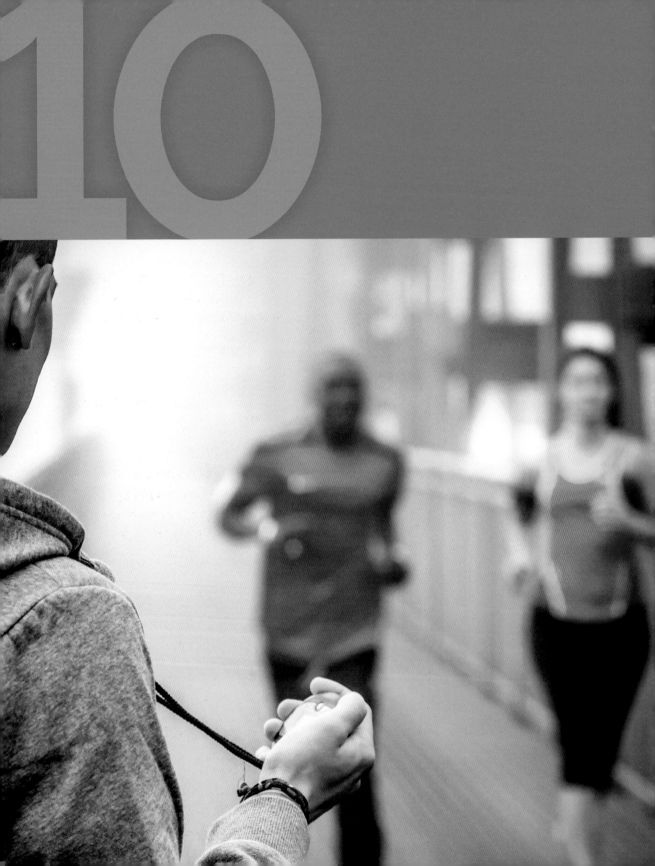

10

PROGRAMME DESIGN CHECKLIST

■ **To achieve consistent results** you need to be able to develop a well designed training programme. Use this checklist to guide you and help you pull everything that you've learnt together into a systematic training programme that will ensure you hit your goal.

1. Training Purpose

Establish your training purpose. Always start with the end in mind and then work backwards.

2. Goal Setting

Write down your goals (outcome, performance, process) and make them SMART (Specific, Measurable, Agreed, Realistic, Timed).

3. Needs Analysis

Figure out where you are starting from. Complete your needs analysis, covering the four key areas: lifestyle, fitness, health and performance.

4. Track Progress

Decide what monitoring tools you are going to use to track your rate of change and adaptation (training diary, load lifted, time to complete 5km etc).

5. Structured Programme

Develop a structured periodised programme that divides your training into manageable phases. This will be the blueprint that you'll work from.

MACROCYCLE

The complete plan (the largest Russian doll – the one that conceals all the other layers). The macrocycle is 'THE BIG PICTURE'.

MESOCYCLE

Several continuous weeks of training (typically 4–6) within the macrocycle, where the training programme emphasises the same type of physical adaptations. It can be thought of as the 'monthly plan'.

MICROCYCLE

Typically a 7-day period but can range between 5–10 days. This will be your 'weekly plan', providing you with details of specific training sessions that need to be completed that week.

When working on your plan, you will need to answer the following questions:

- What is your training availability – how often can you actually train?
- What volume of training can you complete, based on your training availability?
- What type of training will you be completing during each training phase?

6. Workout Planning

Start to plan your workouts. For each workout, you will need to manipulate the following training variables.

REPETITIONS

Adjusting the repetitions for a given exercise can be a very powerful stimulus that will boost your training adaptations.

SETS

Inverse relationships exist between sets and reps as well as sets and the number of exercises that can be completed during the course of a workout.

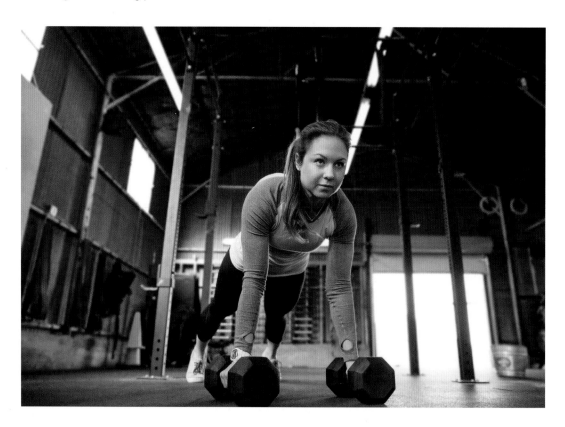

LOAD

How much weight you lift will dictate the speed of movement (tempo) and force production, both of which impact on specific performance outcomes. Typically, there is an inverse relationship between load and repetitions (high load – low reps , low load – high reps).

SPEED OF MOVEMENT

Always programme with 'specificity' in mind to achieve specific training outcomes.

RECOVERY

Your ability to recover between sets is linked to 'available energy'. Once the 'tanks' are empty you can't continue, and to optimise performance, recovery times need to be carefully programmed.

EXERCISE SELECTION

Select the most appropriate exercise, taking into account the level of functionality and how it relates to the performance outcome that you want to achieve.

EXERCISE SEQUENCE

Programme the highest-priority exercises and the most complex exercises early in the training session.

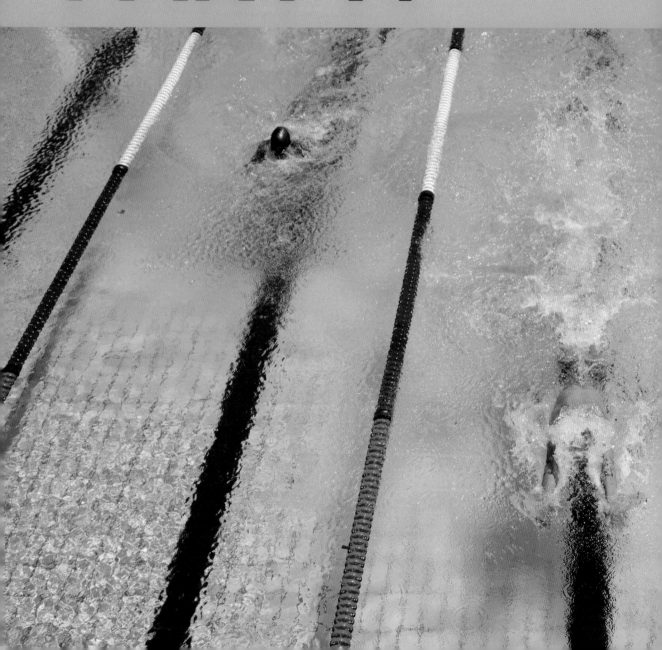

PART IV

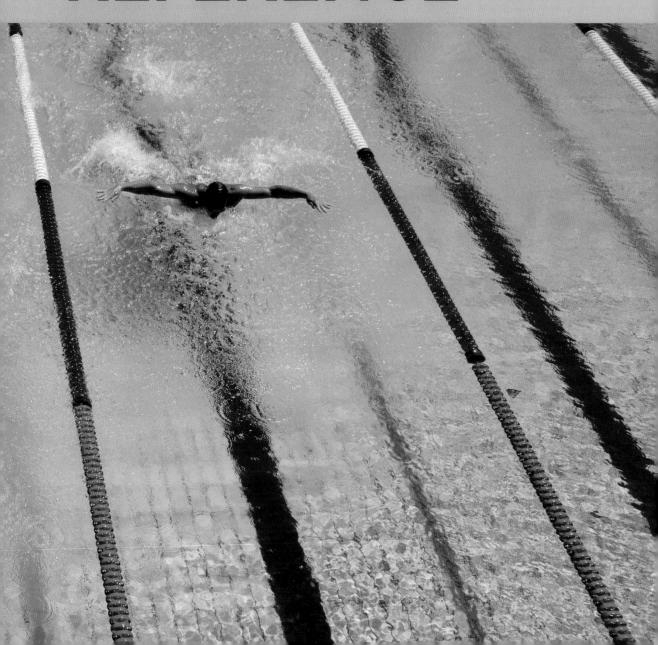

EXERCISE
REFERENCE

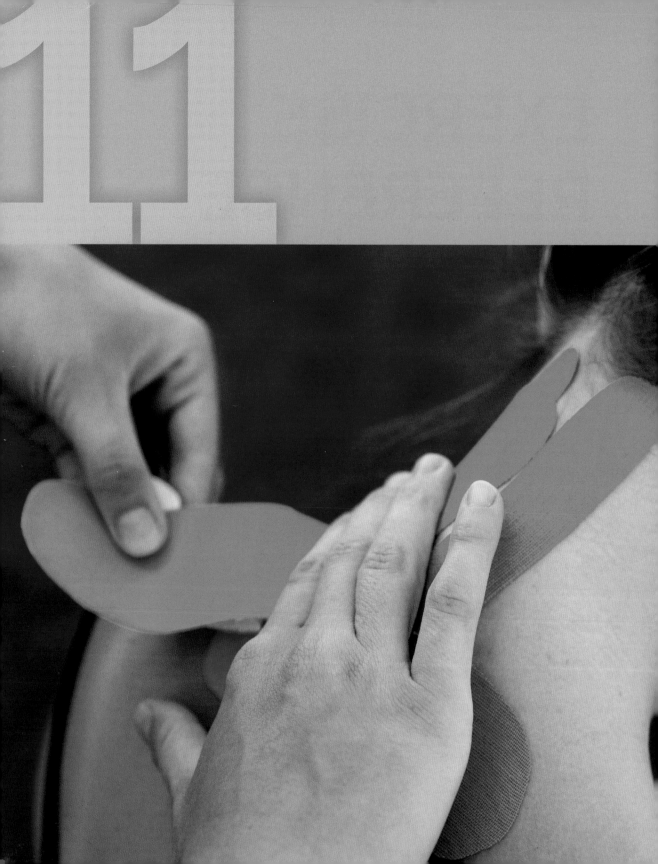

INJURY REDUCTION

■ **Many of the injuries that stop your training** in its tracks can be controlled or prevented if you take action early. In this section I've pulled together a range of exercises that address key injury-prone areas, which I use on a daily basis with the athletes I work with.

LOWER LEG, ANKLE, FOOT

EXERCISE 1: CALF RAISE (GASTROCNEMIUS)

- Stand on the edge of a step, with the balls of your feet firmly planted on the step and your heels hanging over the edge.
- Place your hands against a wall or a sturdy object for balance.
- Raise your heels as high as you can.
- Hold the position for a moment, and then lower your heels back down.

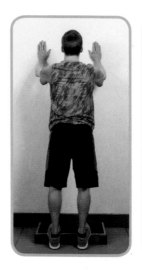
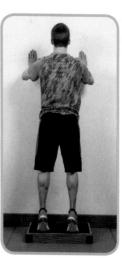

EXERCISE 2: CALF RAISE (SOLEUS)

- Sit on a bench and place your feet on a small step, with the balls of your feet firmly planted on the step and your heels hanging over the edge.
- Raise your heels as high as you can.
- Hold the position for a moment, and then lower your heels back down.

Variations

Work through a full ROM and push evenly through the entire width of your feet when performing both calf exercises. Avoid pushing off from your big toes or the outside edges of your feet. If you want to make these exercises more difficult, reduce your base of support by standing on one leg, add load, or try turning your feet inwards and outwards to work the muscle at different angles.

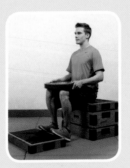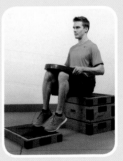

Calf raise (soleus) standing on one leg

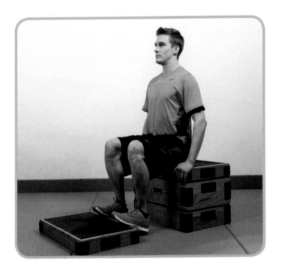

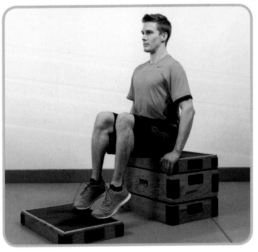

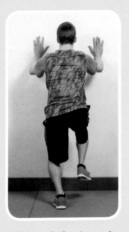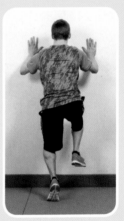

Calf raise (soleus) adding load

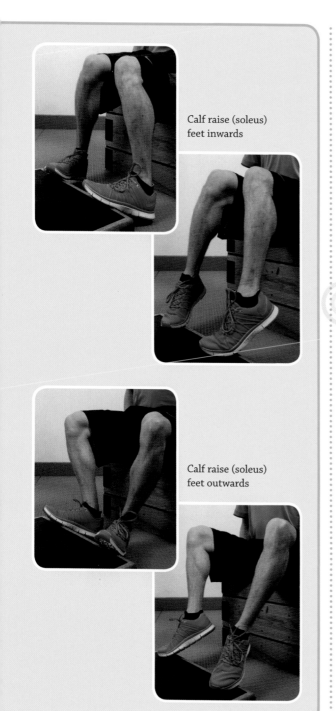

Calf raise (soleus) feet inwards

Calf raise (soleus) feet outwards

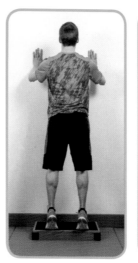 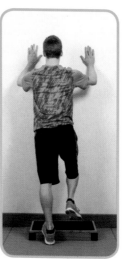

EXERCISE 3: ECCENTRICS

- Stand on the edge of a step, with the balls of your feet firmly planted on the step and your heels hanging over the edge.
- Place your hands against a wall or a sturdy object for balance.
- Raise your heels as high as you can.
- Shift your weight to one foot and slowly lower your heel down.
- Raise your heel and repeat with the other foot.

EXERCISE 4: ANKLE JUMPS

- Stand with your feet hip-width apart and your arms at your sides.
- Shift your weight on to the balls of your feet (raise your toes and imagine you've slid a credit card under your heels – you're now on the balls of your feet).
- Using only your ankles, jump repeatedly.
- Be sure to fully extend the ankles on each jump, trying to reach maximum height. Pull your feet up towards your shins while in the air.

Try these three progressions:

1. **Forward** – Perform the same movement but direct the forces slightly forwards on each jump.
2. **Lateral** – Using the same movement, jump vertically but side to side – make sure you land on both feet at exactly the same time.
3. **Zigzag** – Combine the forward and lateral movements to move forwards in a zigzag pattern.

Once you've mastered Ankle Jumps, you can progress to performing the same exercises on one leg – Ankle Hops

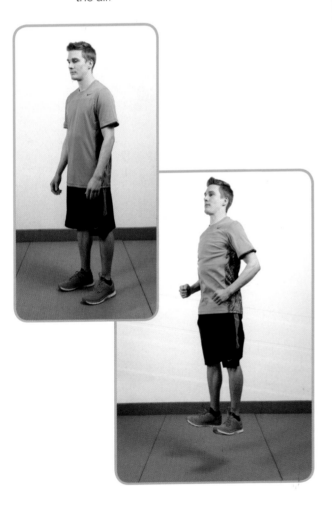

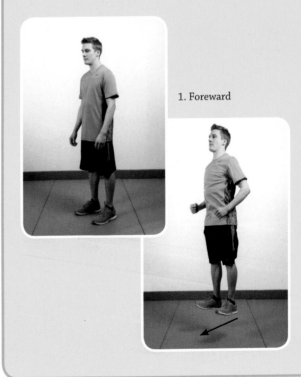

1. Foreward

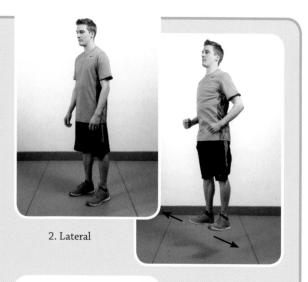

2. Lateral

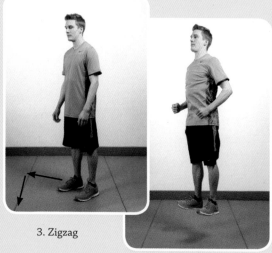

3. Zigzag

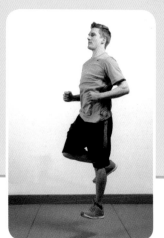

Ankle Hops

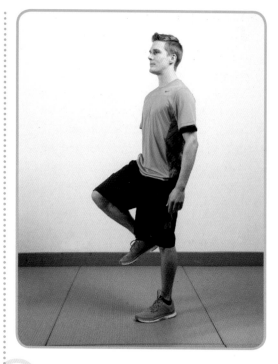

EXERCISE 5: SINGLE-LEG BALANCE

- Stand on one leg, without any support.
- Maintain balance (avoid bracing with the raised leg; hopping; foot touching the floor, or the arms touching something for support).
- Repeat on the other leg.

EXERCISE 6: ANKLE DROPS

- Stand on the edge of a step, with the balls of your feet firmly planted on the step and your heels hanging over the edge.
- Place your hands against a wall or a sturdy object for balance.
- Raise your heels as high as you can.
- Hold the position for a moment, and then 'drop' your heels down quickly, stopping just before you reach the bottom position.

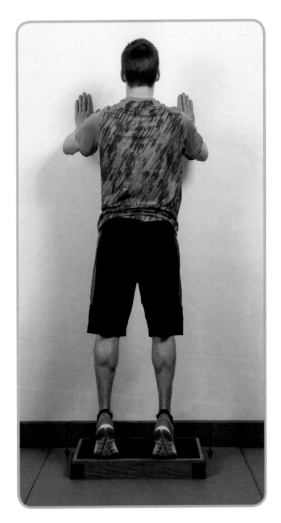 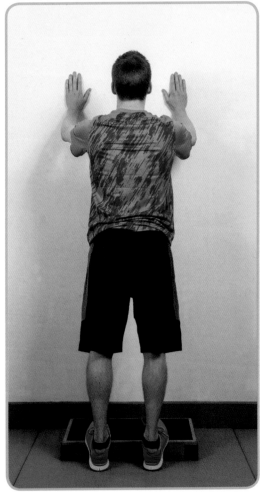

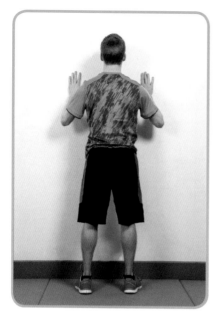

EXERCISE 7: ECCENTRIC KNEE SQUAT

- Stand facing a wall, feet shoulder-width apart, toes just a few inches from the wall. Touch the wall lightly for support.
- Bend at the knees, keeping your torso upright, so that your knees lightly touch the wall.
- Return to the starting position.
- Repeat, but point your knees to the left as you move towards the wall. Keep the hips facing forwards.
- Return to the starting position.
- Repeat, but point your knees to the right as you move towards the wall.
- This sequence (front, left, right) represents 1 rep.

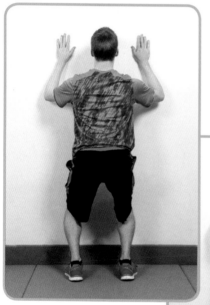

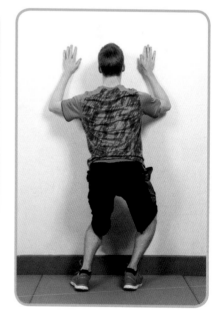

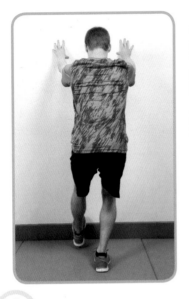 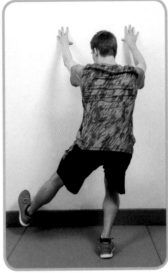 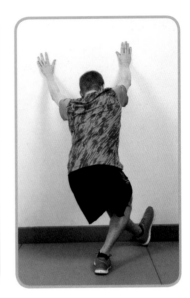

EXERCISE 8: ECCENTRIC REACH

- Stand facing a wall, an arm's length away. Touch the wall lightly for support.
- Stand on your right leg, with your left leg relatively straight with the foot just off the floor and positioned towards the front of your body.
- Bend your right knee and move the left foot towards the wall until it touches.
- Return to the starting position.
- Complete the same movement but moving the left foot towards the left until it makes contact with the wall.
- Return to the starting position.
- Complete the same movement but moving the left foot towards the right until it makes contact with the wall.
- Return to the starting position and repeat with the other leg.
- This sequence (front, left, right) represents 1 rep.

EXERCISE 9: DYNAMIC ACHILLES STRETCH

- Stand facing a wall, an arm's length away.
- Stand on your right leg with the knee slightly bent (as it would be during the stance phase of running).
- Place both hands on the wall for support.
- Rock forward towards the wall until you feel a stretch in your right calf and Achilles. Hold for 20 seconds.
- Roll your foot towards the inside and hold for 10 seconds, then roll your foot towards the outside and hold for 10 seconds.
- Repeat with the other leg.

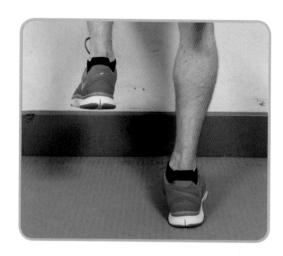

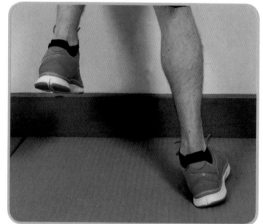

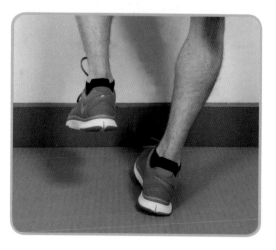

Athletic position

This is the starting position for many exercises. It involves standing with the feet hip-width apart with the hips, knees and ankles slightly bent.

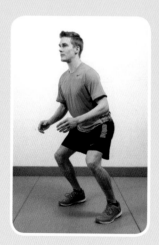

KNEE

EXERCISE 10: MINI-BAND
LATERAL STEP

- Loop a mini-band just above your ankles
  and drop into an athletic position (triple
  flexion at the hips, knees and ankles).
- Leading with the left knee, step laterally.
- Bring the right foot to the left.
- Repeat, stepping to the left.

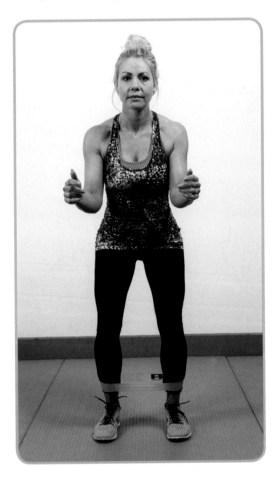
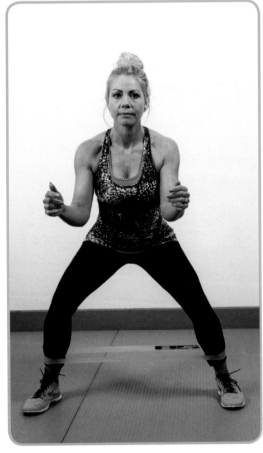

Variations

There's a huge variety of drills that can be performed using the mini-band.

1. **Tall** – Instead of adopting an athletic position, stand up tall – it will feel like a completely different exercise.
2. **Offset** – Drop into an athletic position but this time split your feet so that you're in an offset stance.
3. **Diagonal** – Sit into an athletic position and step diagonally forwards with the right leg, then repeat with the left. You can also perform this exercise stepping diagonally backwards.
4. **Box** – My all-time favourite mini-band drill because it combines a range of movements – perfect for when time is tight. Adopt an athletic position and then complete the following sequence:
   - 2 lateral steps right
   - 1 diagonal step forwards with the left leg
   - 1 diagonal step forwards with the right leg
   - 2 lateral steps left
   - 1 diagonal step backwards with the right leg
   - 1 diagonal step backwards with the left leg

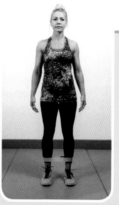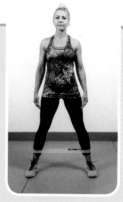

1. Tall

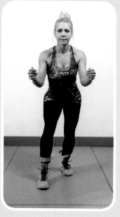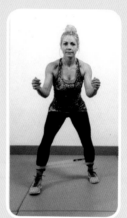

2. Offset

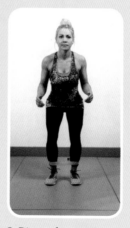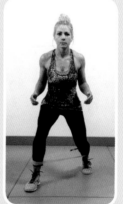

3. Diagonal

EXERCISE 14: 4-POINT HIP EXTENSION

- Adopt a 4-point kneeling position (on all fours), maintaining a flat back.
- Contract your glutes, extend the left hip and leg and hold for a count of 3–5 before changing sides.
- Avoid any movement through the lower back.

This is a great exercise that is often overlooked as simply being something that would crop up in a legs, bums and tums class. It teaches you how to recruit the gluteals while maintaining a stable torso (many of you reading this book will have gluteal amnesia – your bum has forgotten what it is supposed to do and kind of just sits there doing very little – which is not particularly useful when you consider that strong glutes will help many athletic movements).

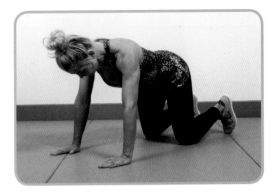

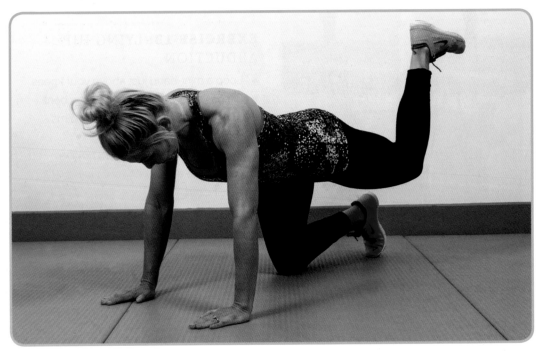

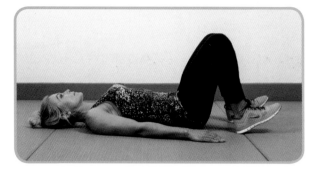

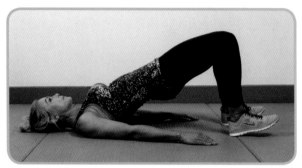

EXERCISE 15: BRIDGE

- Lie flat on your back, arms out to the side, palms facing down.
- Bend your knees to approximately 45-degrees and place your heels on the floor.
- Contract your glutes and hamstrings and raise your hips until they are fully extended.

Variations

If you want to make this exercise more difficult, reduce your base of support by bringing your arms in and crossing them over your chest. You can also take it up another level by marching, either by keeping the knee bent and initiating the movement from the hip or by keeping the hips stable and marching using knee extension.

Bridge: crossing arms across chest

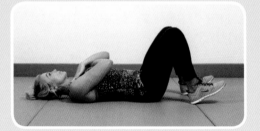

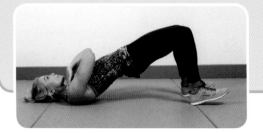

Bridge: marching

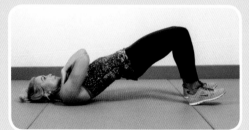

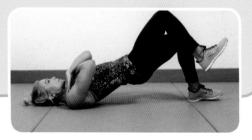

EXERCISE 16: 3-POINT BRIDGE

- Get into the same starting position as for the bridge.
- Raise one foot off the floor and hold for 3–5 seconds.
- Return the foot to the floor and repeat with the other foot.
- Work hard to maintain hip alignment.

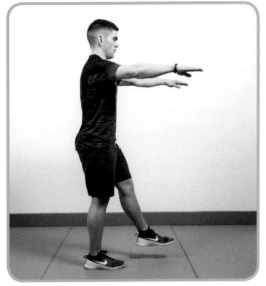

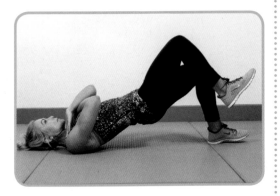

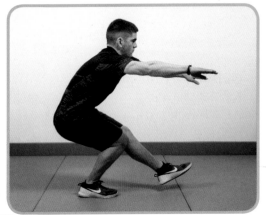

EXERCISE 17: SINGLE-LEG SQUATS

- Stand with your feet hip-width apart, arms by your sides.
- Extend one leg in front of you at about a 45-degrees angle.
- Lower yourself into a squat position (work to a ROM that allows you to maintain correct technique). Allow your arms to extend in front of you (this will help with balance).
- Return to the starting position and repeat with the other leg.

Variations

The single-leg squat is something of an endangered species in local gyms and health clubs. Not because they don't work, but because they are tough! Single-leg strength is one of the most important qualities in performance training and there's clear evidence to link improved lower-limb strength with enhanced speed, power output, running economy and time to exhaustion for a wide range of sports. If you don't have single-leg squats as part of your programme, then you're missing out on a vital component of your overall training.

If this is too tough, take the exercise back a couple of steps and start with Single-Leg Bench Get-Ups or Partial Single-Leg Box Squats as illustrated here. Both exercises help you develop single-leg strength in a controlled range.

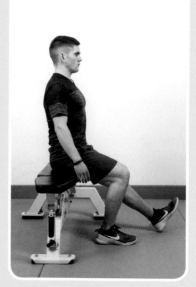 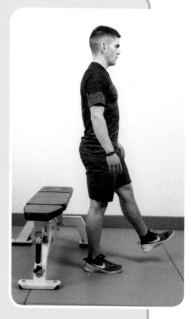

Single-leg bench get-ups

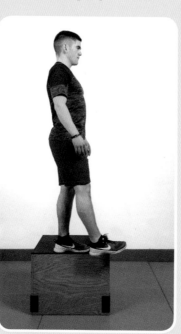 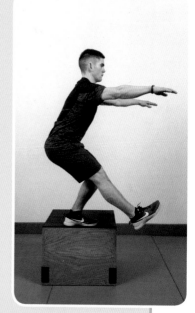

Partial single-leg box squats

SHOULDER

EXERCISE 18: SHOULDER CIRCLE

- Stand with your feet approximately shoulder-width apart, with both arms fully extended above your head so that the biceps almost touch your ears.

- Move the arms in a circular pattern using controlled swings for the desired number of repetitions.
- Make sure the circles are large and take the joint through a full ROM.
- Change direction and repeat.

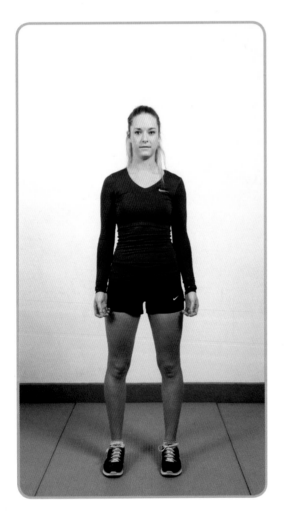
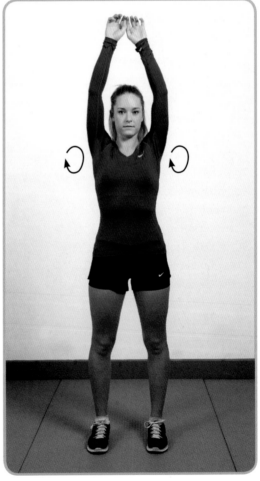

EXERCISE 19: PNF DIAGONAL

- Stand with your feet approximately shoulder-width apart and your arms extended in a diagonal pattern (right arm – high, left arm – low. Make sure the thumb on the right hand points up and the thumb on the left hand points down.
- Switch positions of the arms so that the right arm travels across the body and down and the left arm travels across the body and up.

- The thumb on your left hand should now point up and the thumb on the right hand should now point down.
- Repeat the movement using controlled swings for the desired number of repetitions before changing sides.

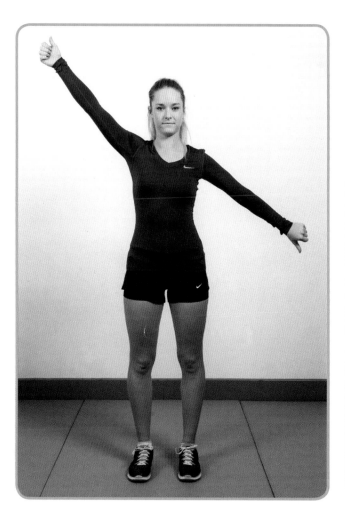

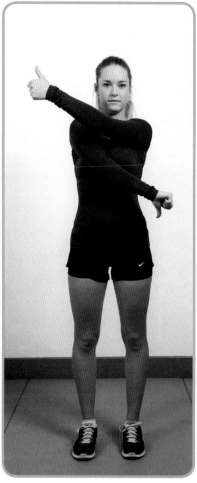

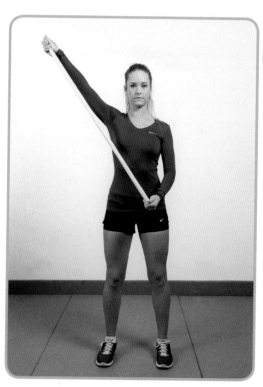

EXERCISE 20: FIGURE 8

- Stand with your feet approximately shoulder-width apart, holding both ends of a stick so that it crosses your torso in a diagonal pattern (right arm – high, left arm – low).
- Complete a figure-of-eight pattern using controlled swings.
- Keep your back flat and chest up and out throughout the exercise.

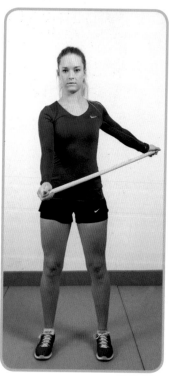
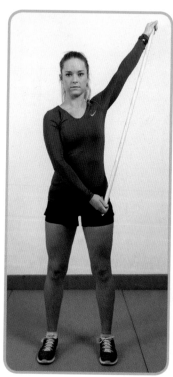
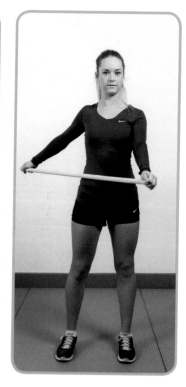

EXERCISE 21: ROUND THE WORLD STRETCH (RTWS)

- Lie on a flat bench, maintaining five points of contact (left foot, right foot, lower back, upper back, head).
- Using two light weights (1.25kg), perform large circular movements clockwise and anticlockwise.

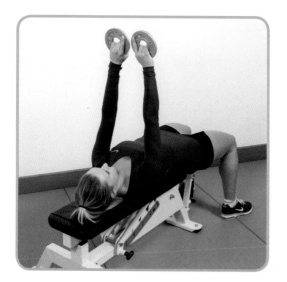

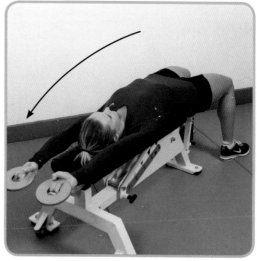

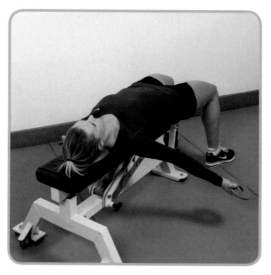

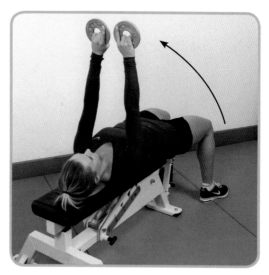

EXERCISE 22: FLUTTERS

- Lie face down on the floor with your arms out to the side.
- Move your arms up and down, making sure you initiate the movement from the scapulothoracic joint (shoulder blades).
- The movement should be small and controlled.

When performing the flutters, make sure you avoid letting the lats take over, pulling the arms down to the sides. Imagine you are trying to squeeze the juice out of an orange that has been placed between your shoulder blades. Try to keep your trapezius as relaxed as possible throughout the movement.

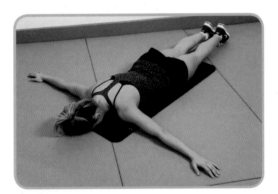

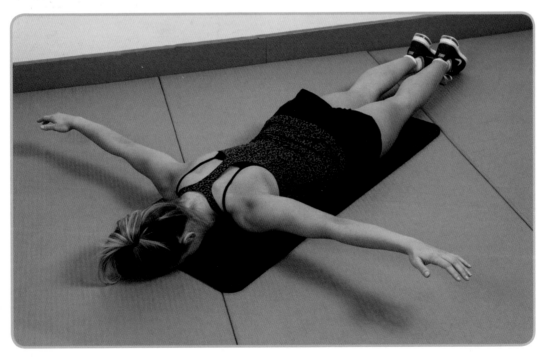

EXERCISE 23: Y T W L

- Lie face down on the floor or on a bench and, using your arms, create the letters 'Y', 'T', 'W' and 'L' in four separate movements.
- Make sure you initiate the movement from the scapulothoracic joint (shoulder blades).
- The arm movements should be small and controlled.
- When performing the 'T', make sure you avoid letting the lats take over, pulling the arms down to the sides.

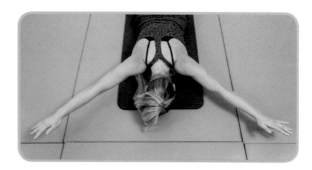

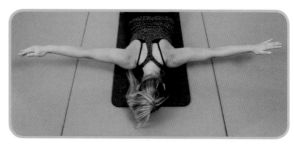

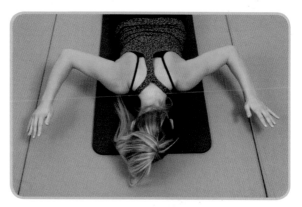

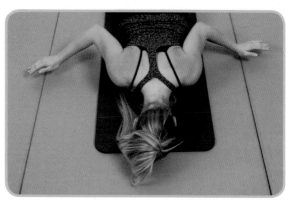

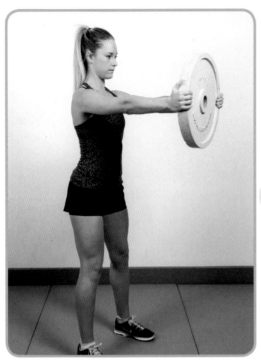

EXERCISE 24: TRUCK DRIVERS

- Stand with your feet hip-width apart.
- Hold a weight at arm's length, with your elbows slightly bent.
- Rotate the weight as far as possible to the right and then back to the left, as if you were turning the steering wheel of a truck.

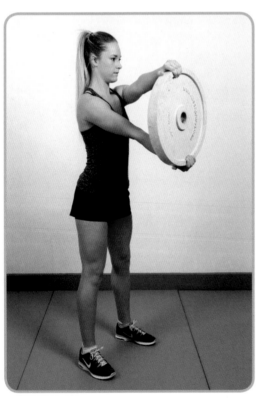

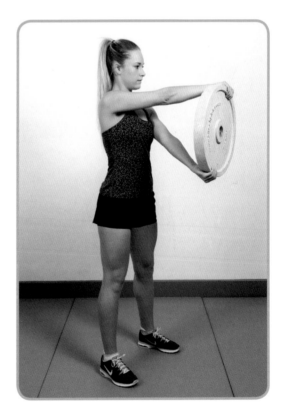

EXERCISE 25: SHOULDER SHUFFLES

- Place a mini-band around your wrists and get into a press-up position.
- Take small steps, moving each hand in a random pattern.
- Try to maintain tension on the mini-band at all times.

Variation

If you find this exercise difficult to do in a full push-up position, simply complete the exercise against a wall.

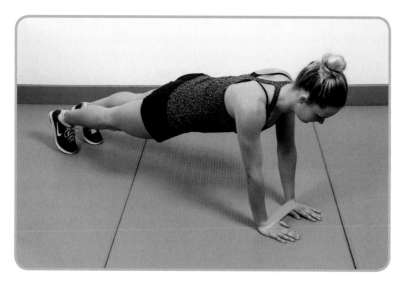

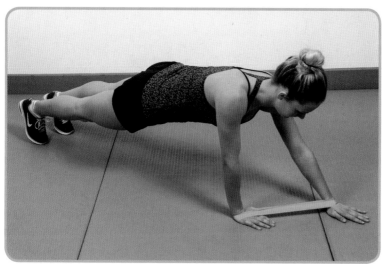

EXERCISE 26: X-BAND WALKS

- Place a superband underneath your feet and, holding on to the ends, cross the band in front of you.
- Holding on to the band, raise your forearms so they are parallel to the floor. Externally rotate your shoulders.
- Retract your shoulder blades.
- While maintaining your posture, take small steps to the right.
- Avoid any unwanted movement through the upper body.

This is an excellent exercise for the shoulder complex but it's also a great conditioning exercise for the upper back and hips.

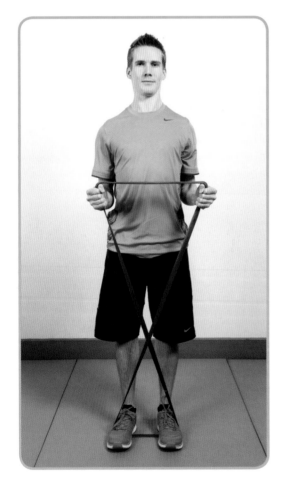

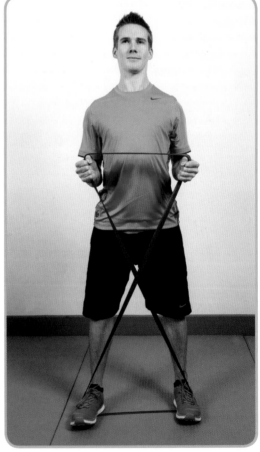

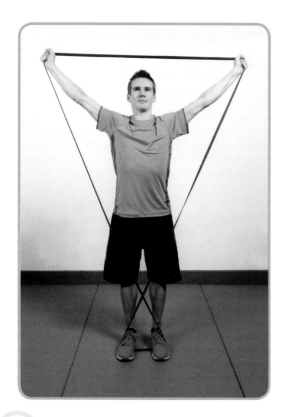 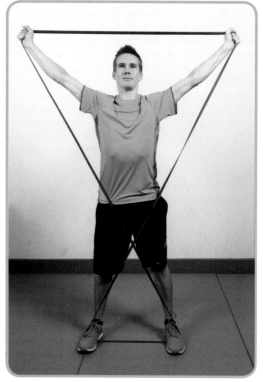

EXERCISE 27: BIG X-BAND WALKS

- Set yourself up as if you are going to perform X-band walks.
- Raise your arms above your head in a Y position.
- While maintaining your posture, take small steps to the right.
- Avoid any unwanted movement through the upper body.

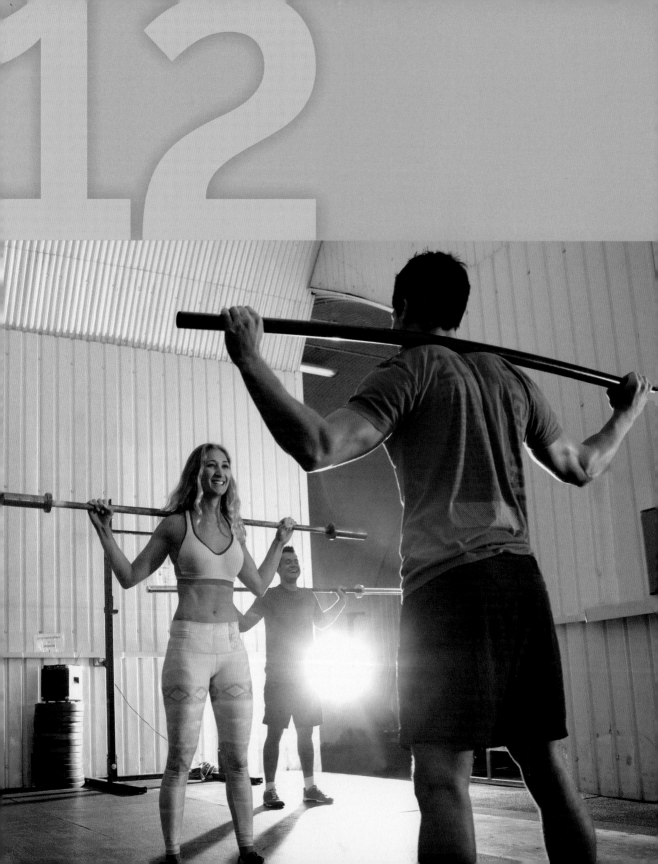

MOVEMENT QUALITY TRAINING

■ **Your body is a highly complex organism** and if you want to be capable of delivering fluid, athletic movements, you need to work on developing gross athleticism. Including MQT sessions in your day-to-day training will reinforce the correct postures and positions of the body in order to allow for effective transfer and expression of force and power.

FLEXIBILITY AND MOBILITY
MYOFASCIAL RELEASE

EXERCISE 28: PLANTAR FASCIA ROLL

- Roll a hockey ball deeply into the plantar fascia on one foot for 2 minutes. Make sure your movements are slow and thorough.
- Repeat on the other foot.

Every athlete I work with performs this simple technique prior to any training session. Limitations at the plantar surface of the foot often correlate with tight hamstrings and lumbar lordosis (curvature of the spine) and rolling a hockey ball deeply into the plantar fascia allows us to start working to correct some of these problems.

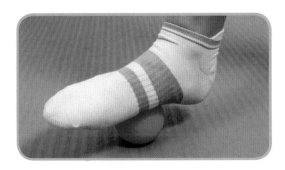

EXERCISE 29: CALF FOAM ROLL

- Sit on the floor with your legs out straight and a foam roll under your right calf.
- Lift your hips off the floor and support your bodyweight on your hands.
- Starting at your Achilles tendon, roll the foam up and down the length of your calf.
- Make sure you rotate your lower leg to hit the lateral and medial portions of the calf.
- Repeat with the foam roll under your left calf.

> If you are finding the single leg version of this exercise too tough, place both legs onto the foam roller.

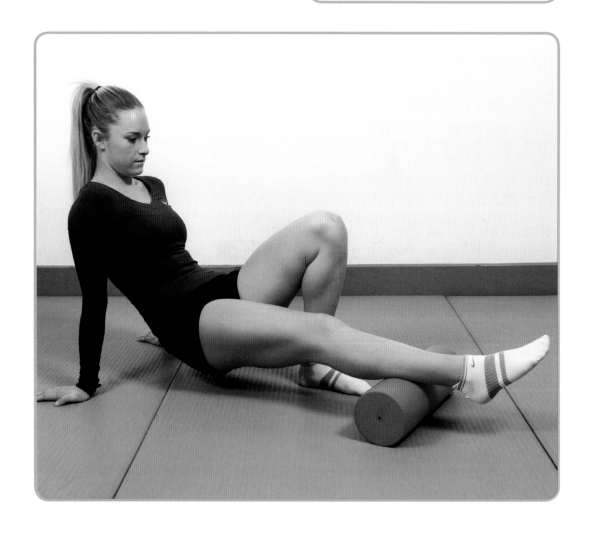

EXERCISE 30: TIBIALIS ANTERIOR FOAM ROLL

- Kneel with a foam roll under your shins and your hands positioned on the floor in front of the foam roll, shoulder-width apart.
- Your hands remain in the same position while you roll up and down the length of your shin.
- Make sure you rotate your lower leg to hit the lateral and medial portions of the shin.

It's a good idea to work on these muscles alongside your calf muscles (gastrocnemius and soleus), as they work together and have important roles to play to during standing, walking and running.

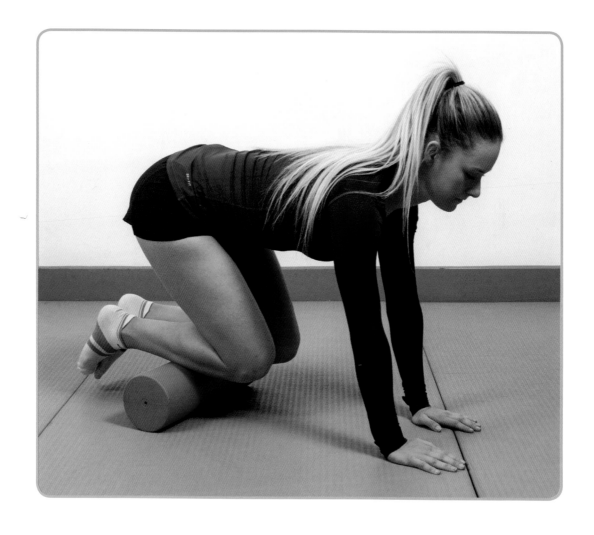

EXERCISE 31: GLUTEAL FOAM ROLL

- Sit on a foam roll.
- Place your right ankle on top of your left knee and pull your ankle towards the shin (dorsiflexion).
- Shift your weight on to the glutes of your right side.
- Roll around your glutes and find those trigger points!

Your glutes extend your hips and trunk (really important for running and jumping) so you need to look after them. If you sit down all day, or spend long periods of time sat down in the car or on flights, chances are your glutes are going to be tight and that's going to compromise your athletic potential.

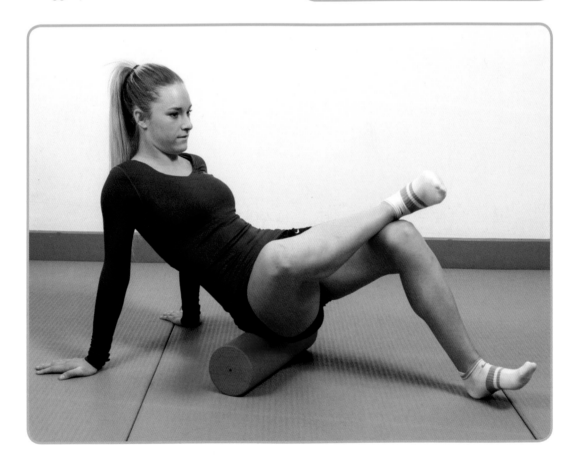

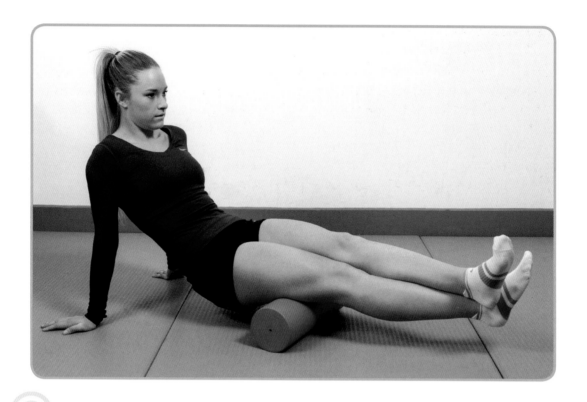

EXERCISE 32: HAMSTRINGS FOAM ROLL

- Sit on the floor with a foam roll under your hamstrings.
- Stack the other leg on top.
- Roll up and down the length of the hamstrings.

You can adjust your body position to target the medial and lateral aspects of the hamstrings.

EXERCISE 33: QUADRICEPS/ HIP FLEXORS FOAM ROLL

- Lie face down on the floor (elbows and forearms forming a triangle, with your fists underneath your forehead). Place a foam roll under your thighs.
- Roll up and down the length of your thighs.
- You can increase the intensity by crossing one leg over the other and focusing on one side.

> If you want to target the medial quadriceps, turn your feet out ... enjoy the 'mild' discomfort! Turn your feet in to hit the lateral aspects.

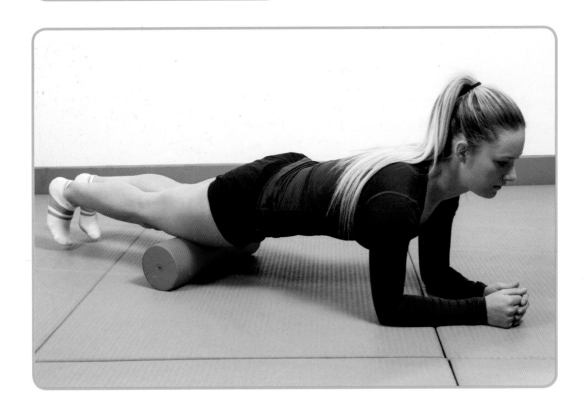

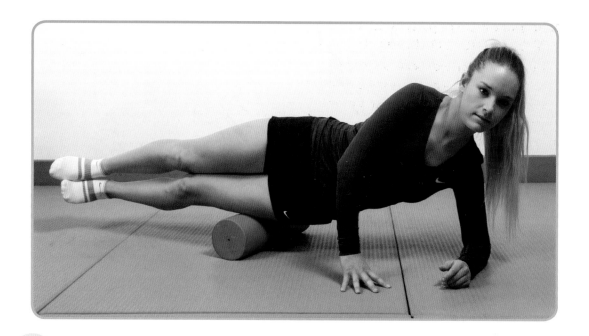

EXERCISE 34: ILIOTIBIAL BAND (ITB) FOAM ROLL

- Lie on your side with a foam roll under your thigh. (You need to keep your top hip 'over'. If you open up, you will drop off the ITB and you won't get the benefit of the exercise.)
- Roll along the length of the ITB from your hip to just above the knee.
- Repeat on the other side.

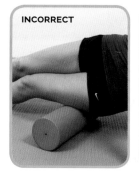

INCORRECT

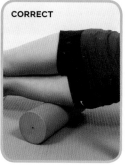

CORRECT

This is probably the one technique that results in a stream of expletives from my athletes. The ITB is usually as tight as a banjo string. A tight ITB can be at the root of many niggly injuries. Don't be tempted to skip this exercise. Your knees will thank you in the long run.

EXERCISE 37: THORACIC FOAM ROLL

- Lie on your back with a foam roll under your mid back.
- Wrap your arms around your body as if you are giving yourself a big hug.
- Roll from your mid back up to your shoulders.

Poor posture is a common problem and if you are desk-bound or sitting behind the wheel of a car for most of the day, the chances are you will have increased thoracic kyphosis (rounded upper back).

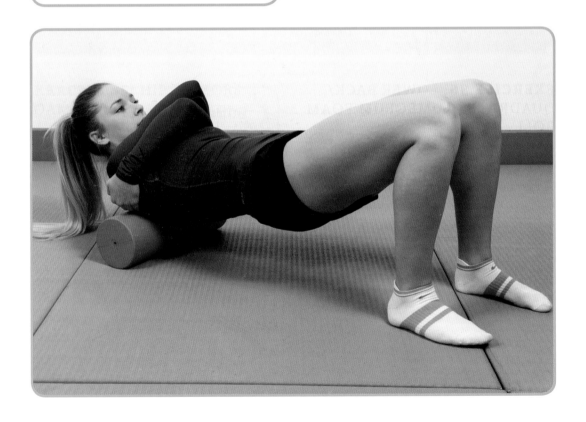

STATIC

All the static flexibility exercises described in this section can be performed statically or dynamically. I've described the static exercises and I would recommend these if you are looking for a more developmental stretch that actually improves ROM. Simply maintain the stretch position for an extended period of time (no longer than 30 seconds), and repeat 2 or 3 times for each exercise. If you want a more dynamic stretch, perform the three-dimensional dynamic variations for which you change the orientation of the limbs every 10–30 seconds.

EXERCISE 38: HAMSTRING STRETCH

- Lie on your back with one knee bent, foot on the floor.
- Bring your other knee towards your chest and hold firmly on to the back of your thigh with both hands.
- Straighten your knee as much as possible, while keeping the thigh close to your chest.

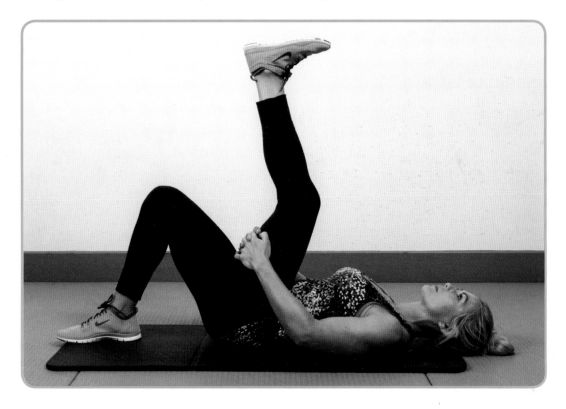

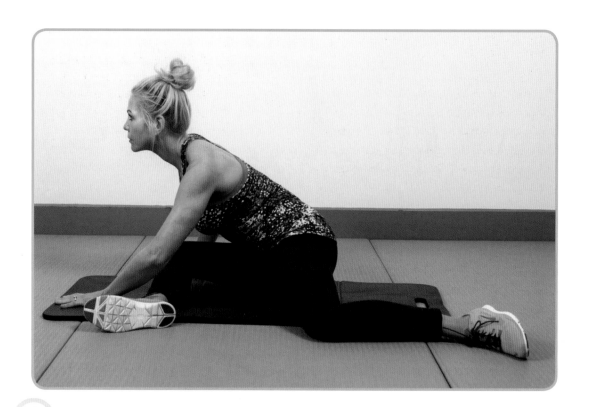

EXERCISE 39: HIP STRETCH

- Sit on the floor with both legs at a 90-degree angle.
- Maintain a flat back position as you walk your hands forwards and feel a stretch in your hip.

 Bend from the hips and not the back

EXERCISE 40: HIP FLEXORS/ QUADRICEPS STRETCH

- Move into a lunge position and drop the back knee to the floor.
- Maintain a slight forward lean in your torso, while shifting your body slightly forwards.
- Place your hands on your hips and push the front of the hip of the back leg towards the floor.
- Repeat on the other side.

> This is a great exercise for getting some length back into chronically tightened hip flexors and quadriceps.

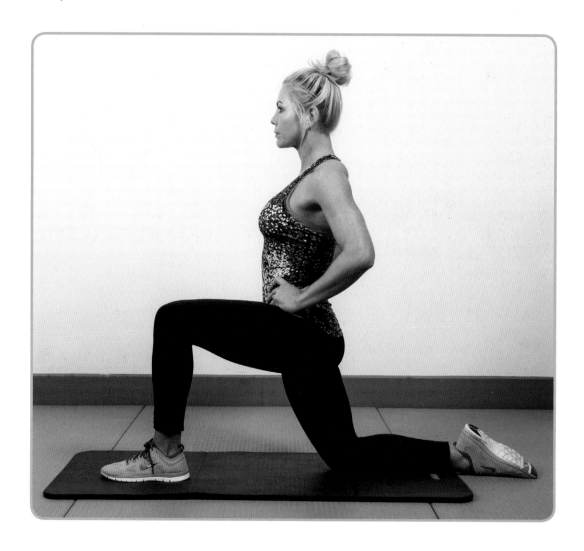

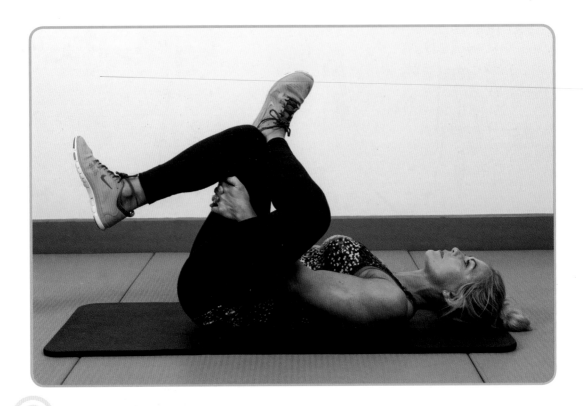

EXERCISE 41: GLUTEAL STRETCH

- Lie on your back with your knees bent at a 90-degree angle and both feet flat on the floor.
- Place your left ankle on your right knee.
- Pull the right leg up towards the chest to feel a stretch down the right gluteals.
- Repeat on the other side.

This is an excellent stretch to work on improving the flexibility and mobility in your glutes and will be of partciular benefit for anyone that spends significant amounts of time sitting down.

EXERCISE 42:
GASTROCNEMIUS STRETCH

- Stand upright about 0.75 metres (2–3 feet) from a wall or stable surface in a split stance.
- Keep the heel of your back foot flat on the floor with the foot pointing straight forwards.
- Bend the front knee, keeping the back knee straight.
- Repeat on the other side.

The gastrocnemius is the powerhouse of the calf muscles and plays an important role in running and jumping activities.

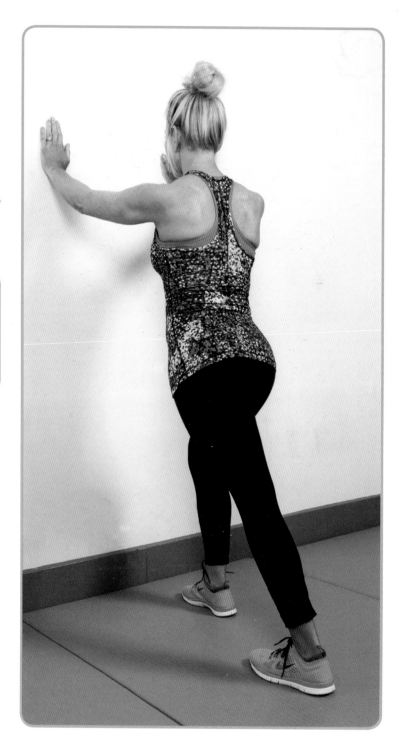

EXERCISE 43: SOLEUS STRETCH

- Stand upright about 0.75 metres (2–3 feet) from a wall or stable surface in a split stance.
- Bend the back knee, keeping the heel of your back foot flat on the floor.
- Repeat on the other side.

The soleus plays an important role in maintaining standing posture and slower more edurance based activities.

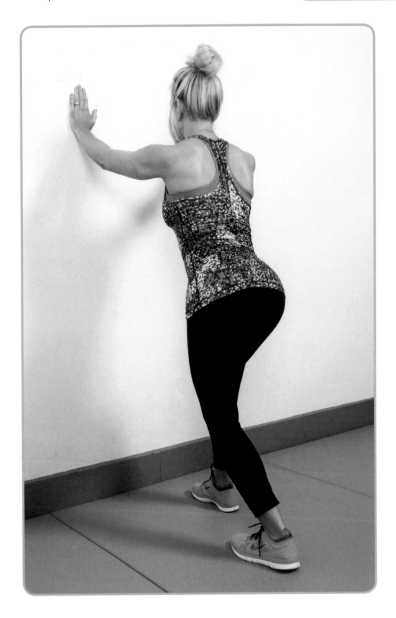

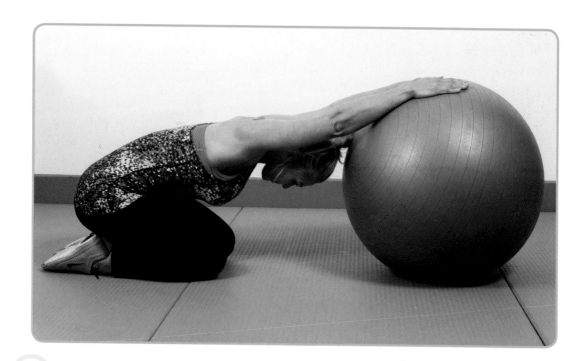

EXERCISE 44: BACK STRETCH

- Place both hands together on top of a stability ball.
- Relax your head down between your arms while sitting your hips back on to your lower leg and ankle.

This stretch targets the muscles in your upper back and shoulders.

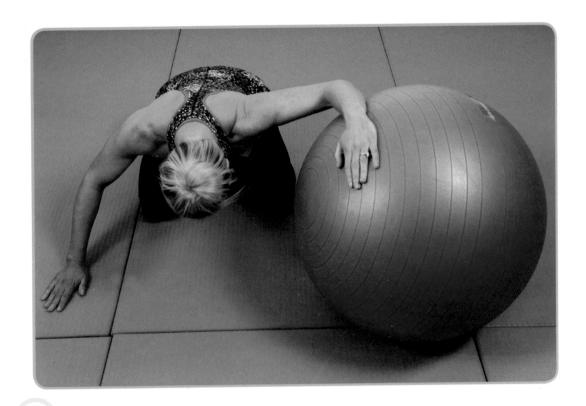

EXERCISE 45: CHEST STRETCH

- Adopt a 4-point kneeling position.
- Place your left arm on top of a stability ball with your elbow bent at 90 degrees.
- Drop your left shoulder towards the floor and feel the stretch across your chest.
- Repeat on the other side.

> You shouldn't feel the stretch in the shoulder.

DYNAMIC

EXERCISE 46: LOW BACK COMPLEX

- Lie on your back and pull both knees into your chest with your hands. Repeat with increasing range.
- Drop your arms to the sides and drop both legs to one side. Lift the legs back to the centre and drop them to the other side. Repeat until you feel loose.
- With your knees dropped to one side, slide out the bottom leg so that it is straight.
- Press the bent top knee into the floor with your hand.
- Repeat on the other side.

> To increase the stretch, slide the bottom leg backwards as far as possible. To increase the stretch further, reach overhead with your free arm.

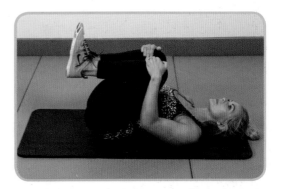

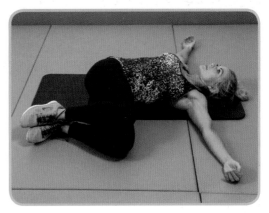

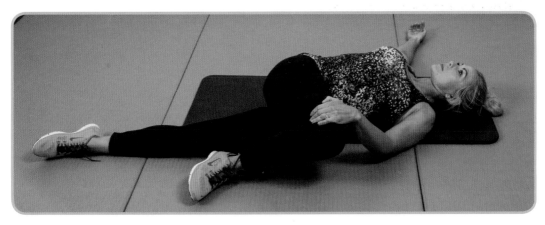

EXERCISE 47: HIP FLEXOR COMPLEX

- Kneel in a lunge position with your right leg back. Keep your chest up and out and your core 'braced'.
- Press your right hip forwards until you feel a light stretch.
- Reach your right arm up in the air and repeat, pressing the right hip forwards.
- Lean your body over to the left side and push the right hip slightly outwards.
- From the leaning position, rotate your torso by turning the chest upwards, reach the right hand upwards and turn the palm to the ceiling.
- Return to the start position and step your left leg out to a side lunge until you feel a stretch.
- Repeat on the other side.

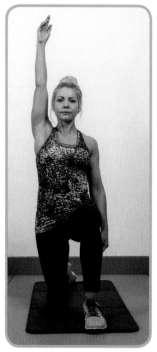
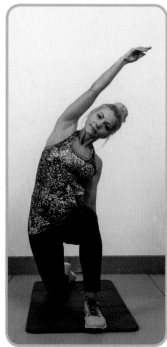
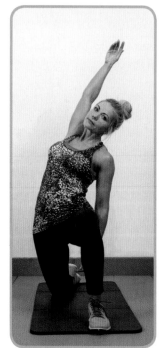
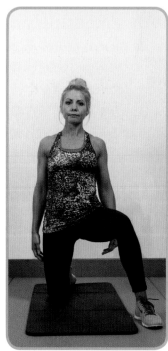

EXERCISE 48: GLUTEAL COMPLEX

- Sit on the floor with both legs at a 90-degree angle and bring your front foot inwards until it touches the other knee.
- Place your hands in front of you in a push-up position, with the arms straight.
- Lower your upper body over the front knee until you feel a stretch.
- Change position slightly so that you move outwards to one side.
- Lower your upper body until you feel a stretch.
- Change position slightly so that you move outwards to the other side.
- Lower your upper body until you feel a stretch.

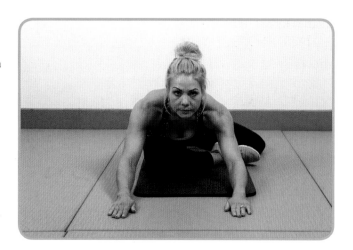

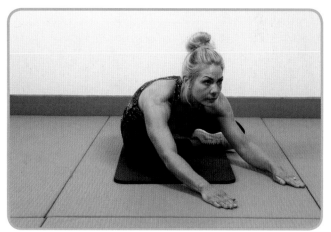

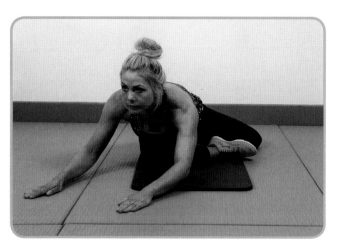

EXERCISE 49:
HAMSTRING COMPLEX

- Lie on your back and bend one leg at a 90-degree angle, placing the foot on the floor.
- Bend the other leg and place your hands behind the thighs. Gently stretch the leg towards the centre of your chest.
- Repeat, moving the leg towards your shoulder.
- Repeat, moving the leg towards your opposite shoulder.
- Repeat on the other side.

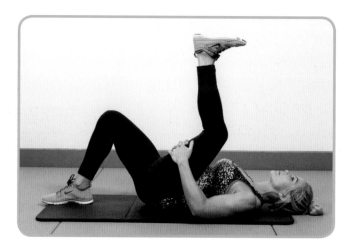

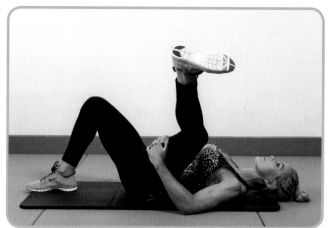

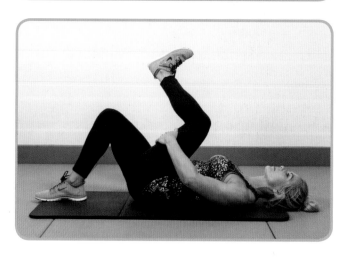

STRENGTH

EXERCISE 50: GIANT CIRCLE

- Stand with your feet slightly wider than shoulder-width apart and your arms extended in front of you.

- Perform squats while circling both arms in a clockwise motion.
- Make sure the circles are large and take the joint through a full ROM.
- Repeat, circling both arms in an anticlockwise direction.
- It is important to keep your head and chest up, maintaining a flat back and weight through the heels, when performing the giant circle.

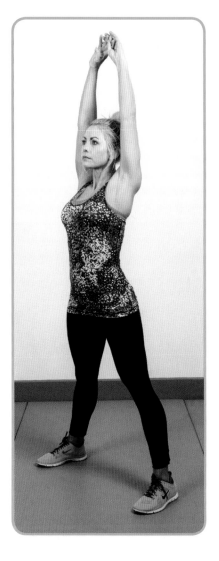

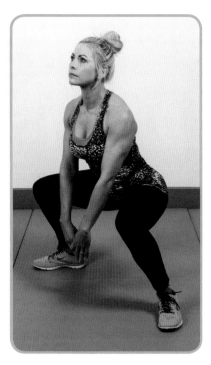

EXERCISE 51: ROMANIAN DEADLIFT

- Stand with your feet approximately shoulder-width apart, with your knees slightly flexed and your feet pointing directly forwards.
- Place your hands behind your head and, maintaining a flat back, bend forwards at the waist towards the floor.

- Extend the hips to return to the upright starting position.
- Keep your back flat and your knees slightly flexed throughout the exercise.

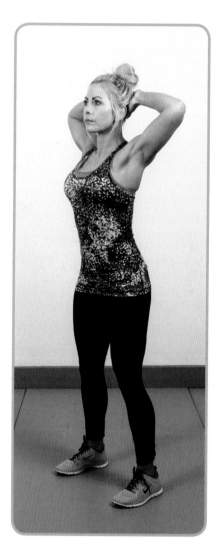 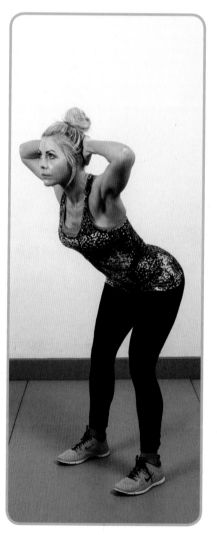

EXERCISE 52: SQUAT

- Stand with your feet approximately shoulder-width apart, with your feet either pointing forwards or in a '10 to 2' position.
- Flex your ankles, knees and hips and lower your body until your thighs are parallel to the floor.
- Extend the hips and knees to return to the starting position.

- Keep your back flat and chest up and out throughout the exercise.

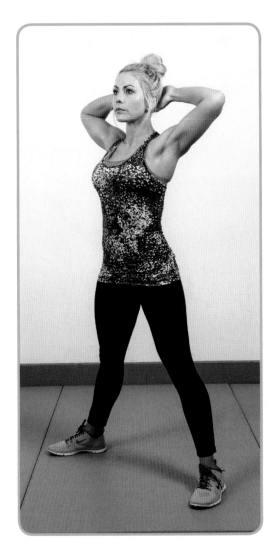

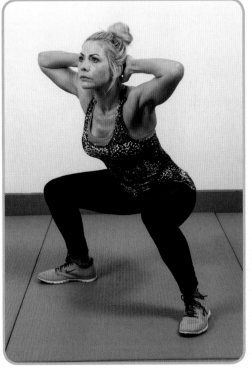

EXERCISE 53: LUNGE

- Stand with your feet approximately shoulder-width apart and pointing forwards.
- Step into a lunge position, creating a 90-degree angle at the front knee.
- Do not allow your back knee to touch the floor and avoid any flexion at the waist.
- Reverse the movement to return to the start.

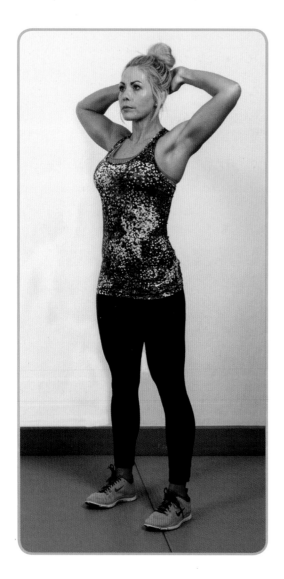
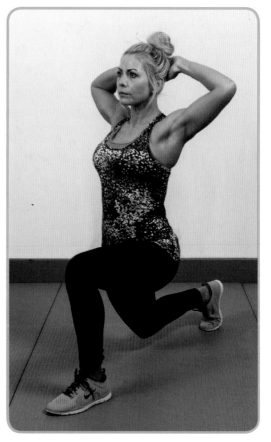

BODY CONTROL – CORE
CORE STABILITY AND STRENGTH – LOCAL STABILISATION

EXERCISE 54: PLANK

- Lie face down, with your elbows and toes taking your weight (position your elbows under your shoulders).
- Keep your ankles, hips and shoulders in line.

- Maintain your back, head and body in a neutral position – squeeze your glutes together, tighten your abdominal muscles to prevent your hips from sagging and brace your shoulders to take the load.

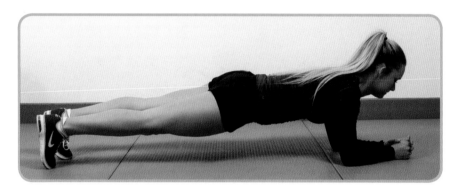

Variations

This simple exercise has many variations that you can use to increase the level of difficulty. Try performing the exercise with two or three points of contact; moving objects placed in front of you; or marching (raise one foot off the floor and hold for 3–5 seconds, then lower the foot and repeat on the opposite side).

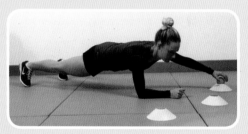

Plank: moving objects

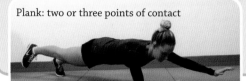

Plank: two or three points of contact

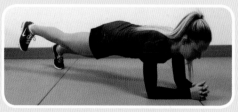

Plank: marching

EXERCISE 55: SIDE HOLDS

- Lie on your side, legs straight, feet stacked one on top of the other.
- Support yourself on your elbow, keeping it in line below the shoulder, and place your free hand on your hip.

- Balance on the side of your stacked feet – squeeze your glutes and tighten up through your stomach.
- Don't allow your hips to drop towards the floor.

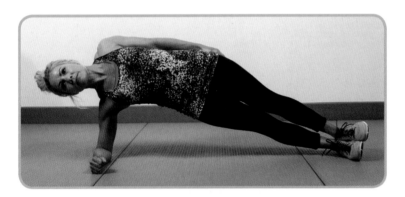

Variations

There are many ways to add some variety to this humble exercise.

1. Rest on the elbow and knees (easier).
2. Stagger your feet forwards and back to add stability (easier).
3. Stack your feet one on top of the other and then lift up the top foot a few inches (harder – enjoy!)
4. Place the hand of the supporting arm on the floor and extend your arm so you are holding the position at arm's length (harder – enjoy!)

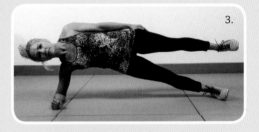

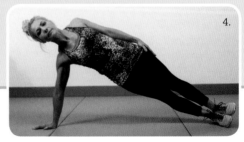

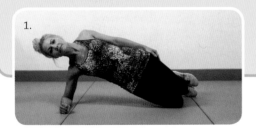

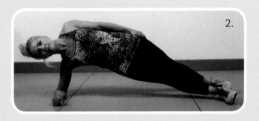

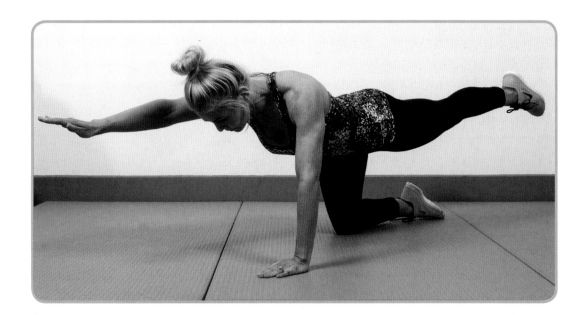

EXERCISE 56: BIRD DOG

- Get into a 4-point kneeling position.
- Lift your right arm and left leg until they are parallel to the floor.
- Hold for 3–5 seconds before returning to the starting position.
- Repeat on the opposite side.

Variation

Once you've mastered the basic exercise, you can make it more challenging by lifting your knees off the floor just a couple of inches. This makes it much harder to control your torso as you switch arms and legs.

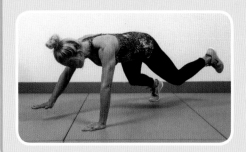

EXERCISE 57: BAND/CABLE ISOMETRICS

- Adopt an athletic position (triple flexion: hip, ankle and knee).
- Take hold of a superband anchored securely at the other end.
- Extend both arms straight out in front of your body, avoiding any rotation through the torso.

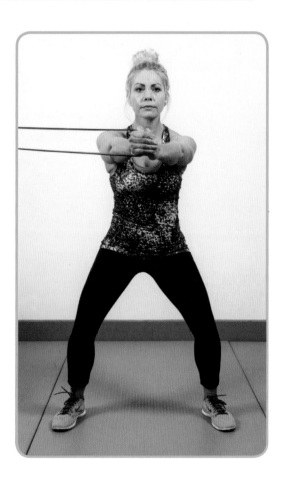

We often forget to train our bodies to avoid 'rotation' but this is a really important quality so I like to have my athletes perform a range of isometric holds to encourage the development of 'anti-rotational' strength.

EXERCISE 58: BARBELL ROLL OUT

- Kneel on the floor and take hold of a barbell loaded with 5–10kg on each side.
- Slowly roll the barbell forwards in a straight line, allowing your hands to move out in front of your body.

- Maintain your body alignment (straight line from shoulder to knee) and pause at the end position before returning to the starting position.

> This is a challenging exercise because it tests your ability to maintain a stable trunk while the arms are moving.

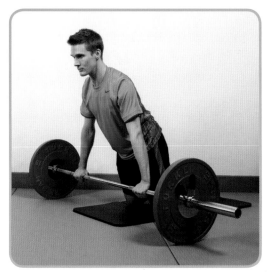

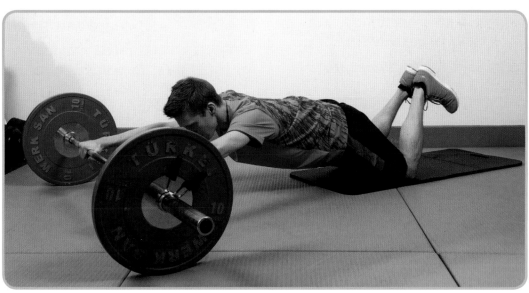

EXERCISE 59: ALEKNAS

- Lie on your back with your hips and knees bent at 90 degrees and your arms fully extended skywards in front of your chest.
- Simultaneously extend your arms and legs fully until they are both close to the floor but not touching it.
- Return to the starting position and repeat.
- The back must remain flat/neutral and your movements must be slow and controlled.

Variation

Maintain a strong and stable core throughout the exercise. Avoid any movement through your trunk, and only move your arms and legs as far as you can without any compensatory movements through the spine. You can increase the difficulty of this exercise by placing a small weight on your shins and in your hands.

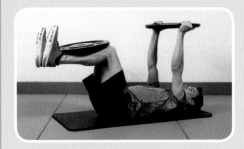

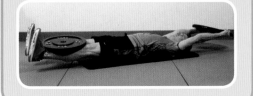

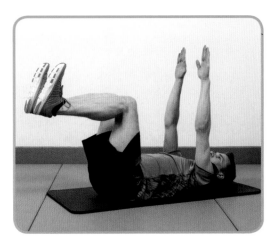

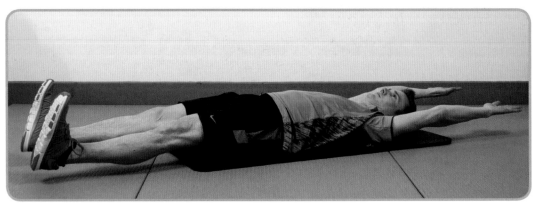

EXERCISE 60: T ROTATE AND HOLD

- The starting position is the same as the top of a push-up, with the arms fully extended.

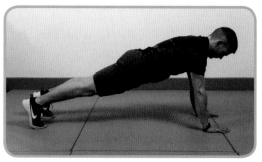

- Take one hand off the floor and rotate your body to the side.
- Hold this position (your body should resemble the letter 'T' with both arms extended), maintaining a stable torso.
- Repeat on the other side.

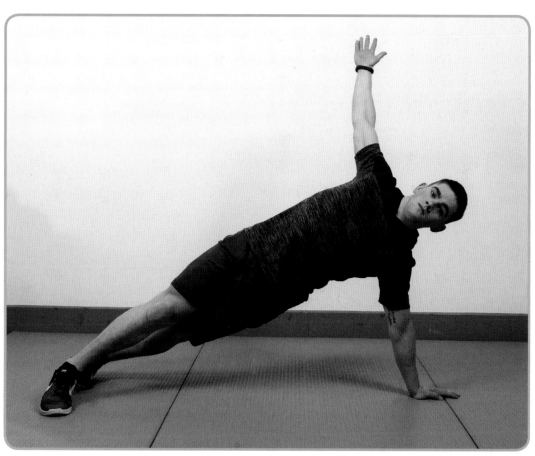

EXERCISE 61: GET-UPS

- Lie on your back with a dumbbell or kettlebell held in your right hand above your shoulder, with your arm straight and vertical. Position your left arm out to the side and bend your right leg so that your right foot is alongside your left knee.

- Pushing off your right foot, roll on to your left hip and up on to your left elbow.
- Push up on to your left hand and, supporting yourself on your left hand and right foot, lift yourself up off the floor.
- Thread your left leg back to a kneeling position, with your left knee and right foot on the floor and the dumbbell or kettlebell locked out overhead in your right hand.
- From the kneeling position, move into a standing position.
- Reverse the movements to come back down to the starting position on the floor.
- Repeat on the other side.

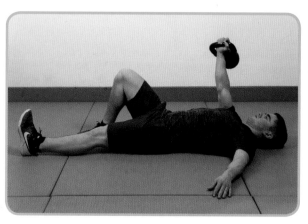

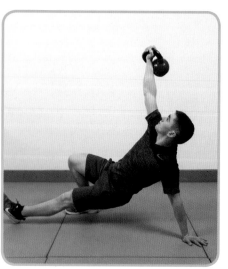

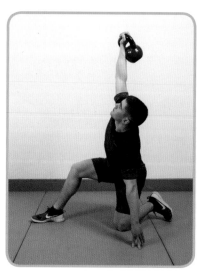

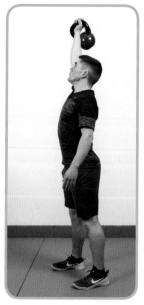

EXERCISE 62: BAND/CABLE ROTATIONS

- Adopt an athletic position (triple flexion: hip, ankle and knee).
- Take hold of a superband that is securely anchored at the other end.
- Rotate the upper body to the right with the arms extended. This is the start/finish position.
- Keeping the arms extended, rotate back to the centre.
- Repeat in the other direction.

Try to keep your hips fixed and facing forwards throughout the movement. Movement should be generated through your core musculature.

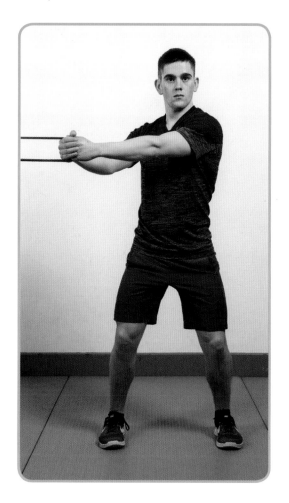
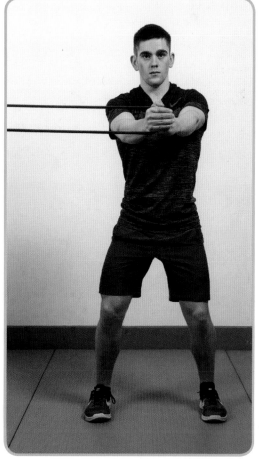

EXERCISE 63: BARBELL ROTATIONS

- Hold the end of a barbell at arm's length and adopt an athletic position, with your feet just wider than shoulder-width apart and a slight forward body lean.
- Rotate to your right as you start to lower the load down towards the outside of your right knee, ensuring your shoulders follow your hands – your left heel can lift from the floor.
- Return to the starting position by forcefully raising the bar back up to the starting position and rotating back to the centre.
- Repeat on the opposite side.

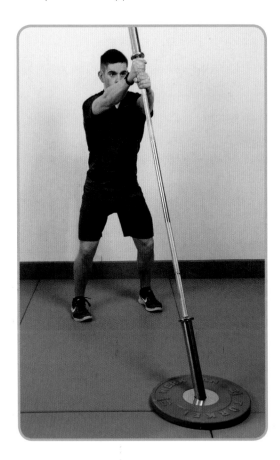
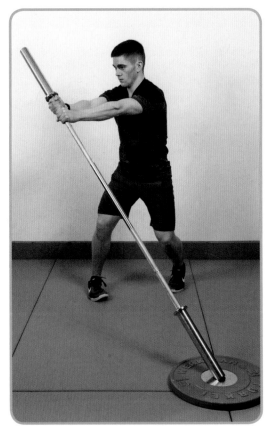

EXERCISE 64: SEATED PLATE ROTATIONS

- Sit on the floor with your knees bent at a 90-degree angle, holding a weight plate in both hands.
- Lean back so that your upper body creates an imaginary V-shape with your thighs.
- Twist your torso to the right side then to the left side in one fluid movement.

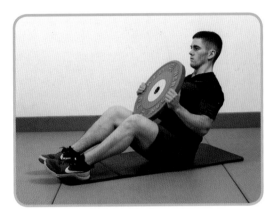

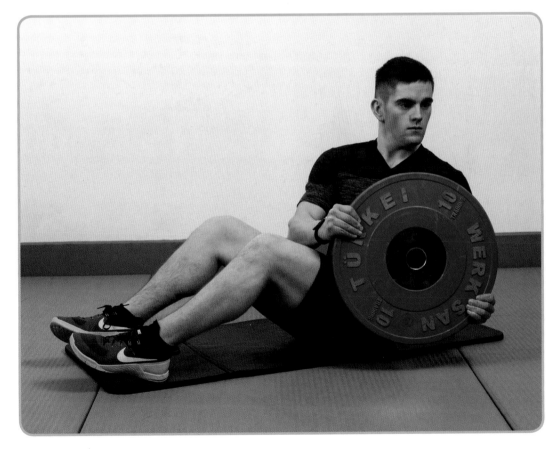

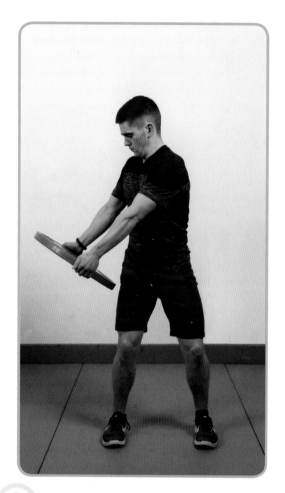

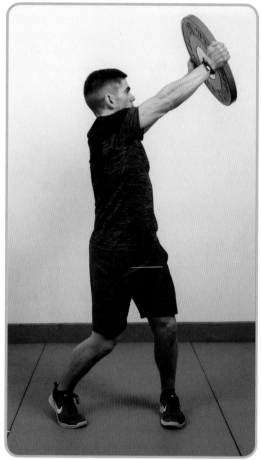

EXERCISE 65: STANDING PLATE ROTATIONS

- Stand in an athletic position holding a dumbbell or weight plate to one side with both hands.
- Drive the weight up and across so you finish with the weight above and behind the opposite shoulder.
- Perform all the repetitions on one side, before moving on to the other.

EXERCISE 66: MEDICINE BALL FRONT ROTATION THROW

- Stand facing a wall and hold a medicine ball at waist level.
- Rotate your trunk to the left, away from the wall.
- Initiate a throw by driving your hip towards the wall followed by your trunk, arms, and the ball.
- Catch the ball with your arms slightly bent before immediately repeating on the same side.
- Repeat on the other side.

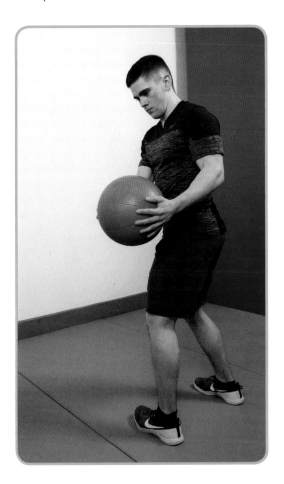
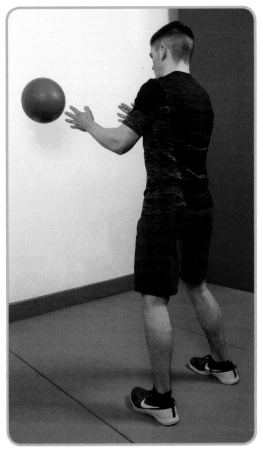

EXERCISE 67: SINGLE-LEG BALANCE

- Stand on one leg with a slight bend in the knee.
- Try to maintain your balance with minimal movement.

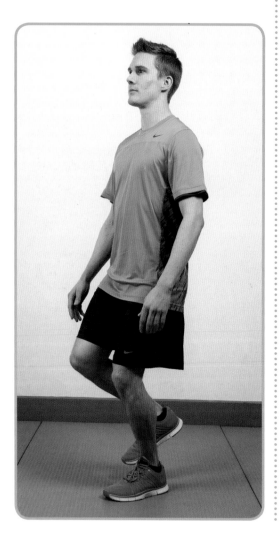

EXERCISE 68: SINGLE-LEG BALANCE AND REACH (FORWARD)

- Stand on one leg with a slight bend in the knee and maintain your balance with minimal movement.
- Extend and point the other leg and toe to the front of your body, keeping your hips facing forwards and level.
- Hold this position for a few seconds, then return to the starting position.
- Try to maintain your balance with minimal movement.
- Repeat on the other side.

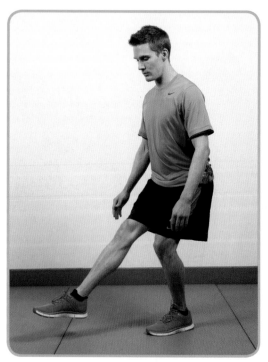

EXERCISE 69: SINGLE-LEG BALANCE AND REACH (BACK)

- Stand on one leg with a slight bend in the knee and maintain your balance with minimal movement.
- Extend and point the other leg and toe behind your body, keeping your hips facing forwards and level.
- Hold this position for a few seconds, then return to the starting position.
- Try to maintain your balance with minimal movement.

Variations

Add an unstable surface (stability disc, beam, half foam roll) to challenge your balance. Add arm and leg movement to make the exercises harder.

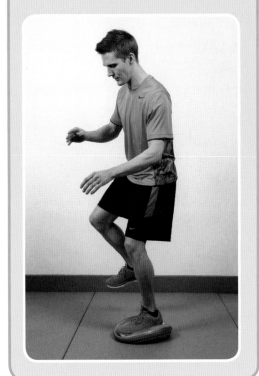

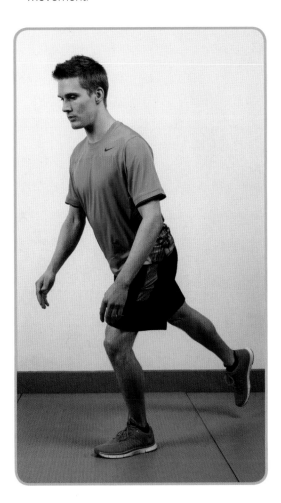

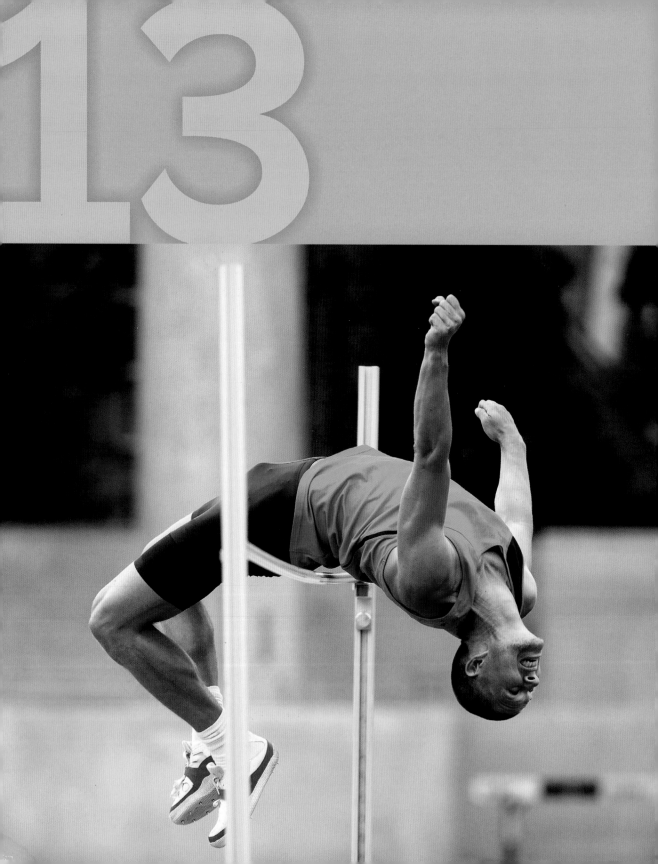

13

STRENGTH AND POWER

■ **The human body has over 660 muscles** (40–45 per cent of its total mass) and when combined with other connective tissues they transmit force to the skeletal system to produce movement. For many years there has been a reluctance to develop strength and power using athletic based resistance-training techniques due to popular preconceptions, myths and old wives tales. However, we know that ignoring strength and power development will stop you unlocking your athletic potential.

KNEE DOMINANT

EXERCISES 70 AND 71: FRONT & BACK SQUAT
Front Squat

- Hold a bar with a clean grip slightly wider than shoulder-width.
- The bar should be racked on top of the anterior deltoids and clavicles, keeping the elbows high.
- Place your feet approximately shoulder-width apart, either pointing forwards or in a '10 to 2' position.

> The front squat is arguably more difficult to learn than the back squat, but the pay-off is that you will develop a great squatting technique with perfect body positioning. It's worth persevering with the 'clean grip', particularly if you want to progress to performing the Clean.

- Flex your ankles, knees and hips and lower your body until your thighs are parallel to the floor.
- Extend your hips and knees to return to the starting position.
- Keep your back flat, elbows high and chest up and out throughout the lift.

Back Squat

- Hold a bar with a closed, pronated grip, slightly wider than shoulder-width. The bar should be racked behind your neck so that it rests on your shoulder muscles – it should not be in contact with your cervical spine.
- Place your feet approximately shoulder-width apart, either pointing forwards or in a '10 to 2' position.
- Flex your ankles, knees and hips and lower your body until your thighs are parallel to the floor.

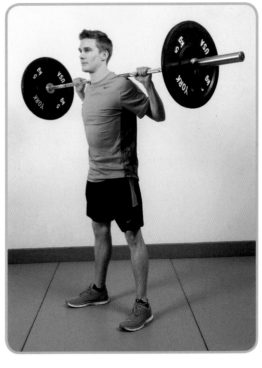

- Extend your hips and knees to return to the starting position.
- Keep your back flat, elbows high and chest up and out throughout the lift.

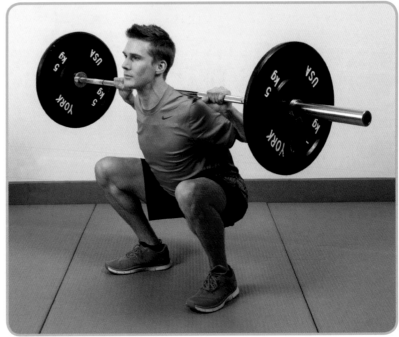

Images show back squat

EXERCISE 72: OVERHEAD SQUAT

- Hold a bar with a 'snatch grip' and raise it overhead, your arms locked at the elbow. Your feet should be flat on the floor, approximately shoulder-width apart, with the toes turned out slightly (at 5 to 1 or 10 to 2, whichever is comfortable). The bar should be aligned with the mid foot throughout.
- When you're ready, bend your ankles, knees and hips to lower your body until your thighs are at least parallel to the floor.
- Keep your chin up, eyes focused straight ahead, and maintain a rigid, but neutral, spine position throughout.
- Pause for a moment in the bottom position, then return to a standing position.

The overhead squat is a demanding exercise but it's a great technique to master. You won't be able to lift significant loads but you'll soon realise that every single muscle in your body is working to maintain that bar over your head.

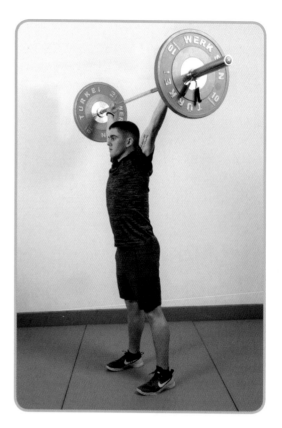

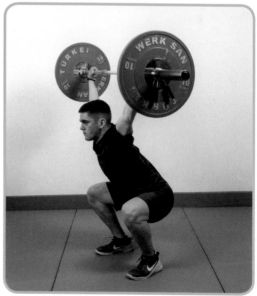

EXERCISE 73: SPLIT SQUAT

- Collect a bar from a rack by resting it on your upper shoulder. Take a stride forwards, so that your front foot is flat on the floor and your back foot is raised on to the toes.
- When you're ready, lower your body into a split squat position by flexing at the hips, knees and ankles.
- Maintain an upright torso throughout, lowering under control so that your bodyweight is evenly distributed between your front and back feet.
- Lower to a position where your back knee is 10cm (4 inches) off the floor, and pause. Your front foot should be flat on the floor throughout the movement.
- Return to a standing position by extending your knees and hips.

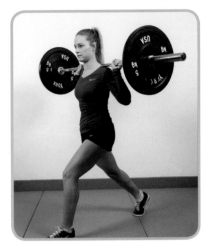

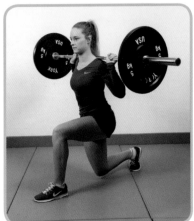

Variation

If you are struggling to master the squat or split squat, use a stability ball to help you work on achieving the correct technique. Place the stability ball against a wall so that it is positioned in the small of your back. The stability ball acts like stabilisers on a bike and allows you to slow the movement down. This provides you with plenty of opportunities to check your technique and ensure that you have proper alignment.

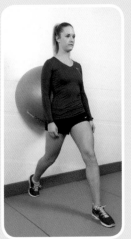

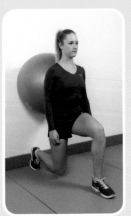

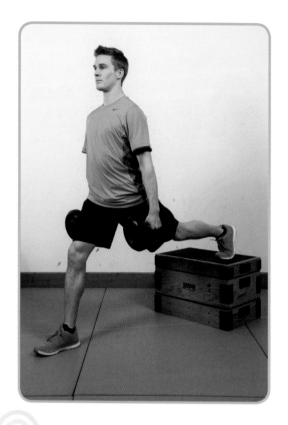

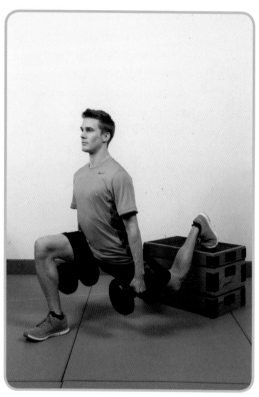

EXERCISE 74: BULGARIAN SPLIT SQUAT

- Place one foot in front of the other with the rear foot placed firmly on top of a bench or box.
- Making sure your front heel remains firmly on the floor, descend as deeply as possible.
- Return to the starting position and repeat.
- Repeat on the other side.

Variations

You can perform the Bulgarian split squat using dumbbells or barbells. The barbell can be placed either in front of your neck or behind it.

EXERCISE 75: LUNGE

- This exercise can be performed using dumbells or a barbell
- Stand with your feet hip-width apart.
- Step one foot forwards as far as possible, landing heel first.
- Descend into the back knee, almost touching the floor before immediately driving up and back to the starting position.

The reverse lunge is great for targeting strength in the glutes and hamstrings as well as developing control through the whole body during dynamic movements.

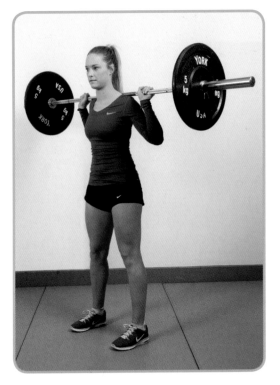

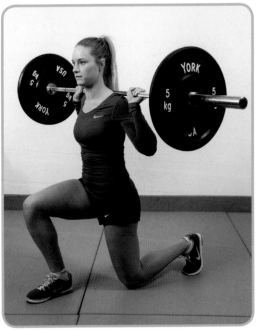

EXERCISE 76: STEP-UP

- Holding a dumbbell in each hand, place one foot on a step box and start the movement by pushing through the heel.
- Maintain an upright torso throughout and avoid 'cheating' by using the rear foot to initiate the movement.
- Finish the movement with the support leg 'locked' and the free leg lifted so that the thigh is parallel to the floor.
- Return to the starting position. Complete the reps on one side before repeating the exercise on the other side.

Not only is the step-up a great exercise to develop single-leg strength but it also challenges your ability to control movement. Use a 30–40cm (12–15½ inch) step box (the height can be changed depending on your height and also your training goal: higher boxes suit power, control and mobility development using lighter loads; lower boxes suit heavier loads to bring about strength gains.

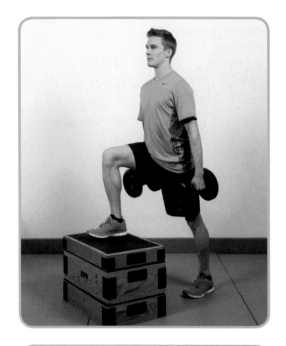

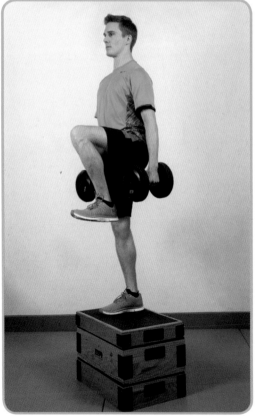

HIP DOMINANT

EXERCISE 77: ROMANIAN DEADLIFT (RDL)

- Hold a bar with a grip approximately shoulder-width wide (your thumbs should brush the outside of your thighs).
- Place your feet approximately hip-width apart, with your knees slightly flexed and your feet pointing forwards.
- Maintaining a flat back position, bend forwards at the waist, lowering the bar towards the floor.
- Extend your hips to return to the upright starting position.
- Keep your back flat, your knees slightly flexed and the bar close to your body throughout the lift.

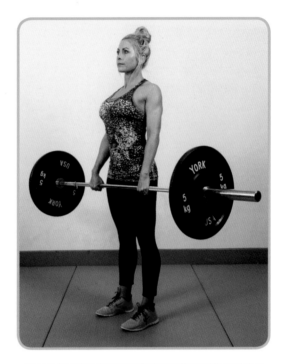

This is a terrific exercise for developing strength and flexibility through the posterior chain. Your ROM will be dictated by your hamstring flexibility, but this will improve over time. The bar should be your 'best friend'; try to keep it as close to your body as possible throughout the lift.

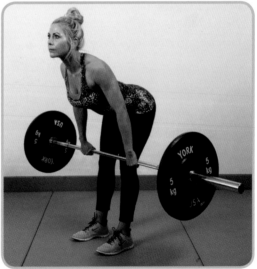

EXERCISE 78: SPLIT ROMANIAN DEADLIFT (RDL)

- Hold a bar with a grip approximately shoulder-width wide (your thumbs should brush the outside of your thighs).
- Place one foot on a small step or a weight plate so that the heel is on the platform and the toes are pointing upwards, with the leg straight.
- Maintaining a flat back position, bend forwards at the waist, lowering the bar towards the floor.
- Extend the hips to return to the starting position. Complete the reps on one side before repeating the exercise on the other side.
- Keep your back flat, your knees slightly flexed and the bar close to your body throughout the lift.

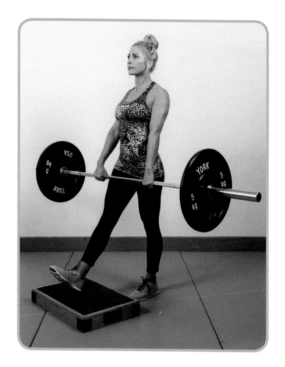

Hip-dominant exercises are neglected in many training programmes, which is a bit daft when you consider their role in running-based activities. Machines traditionally train the hamstrings as knee flexors (non-functional) but hamstrings actually act as powerful hip extensors and stabilisers of the knee. Science has shown that eccentric loading of the hamstrings improves function and decreases injury rate, suggesting that the addition of specific strength training for the hamstrings can be beneficial.

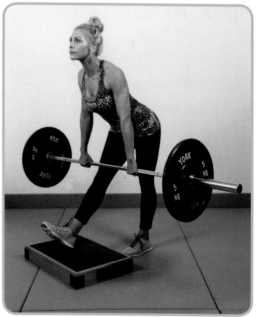

EXERCISE 79: DEADLIFT

- Squat down and hold the bar with a grip approximately shoulder-width wide, outside the knees, with the elbows fully extended. Make sure that your hips are lower than your shoulders.
- Keeping your feet flat on the floor, position the bar just in front of your shins, over the balls of your feet.
- Keep the back flat, chest up and out, shoulder blades together and shoulders slightly in front of the bar.
- Lift the bar from the floor by extending your hips and knees, ensuring the torso-to-floor angle remains constant and your elbows remain fully extended.
- Flex your hips and knees to return to the starting position.

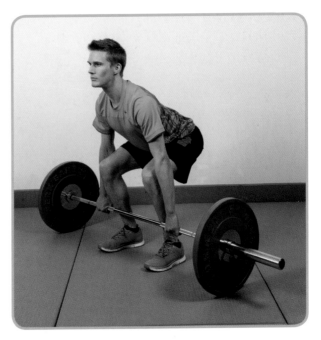

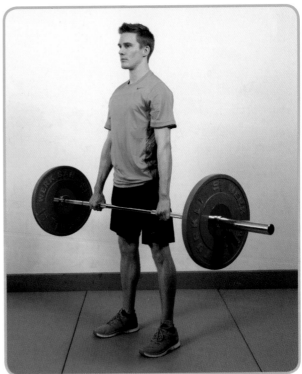

EXERCISE 80: SINGLE-LEG DEADLIFT

- Stand on your right foot with a dumbbell in your left hand.
- Bend both your right knee and hip to sit down into the deadlift position.
- Repeat on the other side.

Some strength and conditioning coaches would refer to this as a hybrid exercise rather than a purely hip-dominant exercise. Regardless of its classification, this is a great exercise for the legs, requiring a significant contribution from the hip musculature.

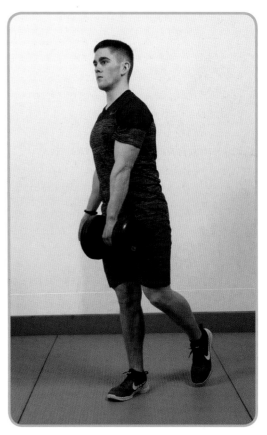

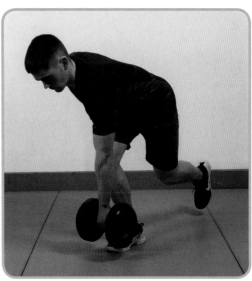

EXERCISE 81: LYING HIP EXTENSION

- Lie flat on your back on the floor.
- Bend your knees to approximately 45 degrees and place your heels on the floor.
- Extend your arms to the side (palms facing down).
- Contract your glutes and hamstrings and raise your hips until they are fully extended.
- Lower your hips until they are about 1cm (½ inch) off the floor.
- Repeat.

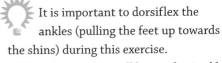 It is important to dorsiflex the ankles (pulling the feet up towards the shins) during this exercise.

- Gluteal activation will be emphasised by lengthening the gastrocnemius to assist the hamstrings.
- Hamstring activation will be reduced, forcing the glutes to do the job they were designed for.
- The foot position relates closely to the foot position in running during heel strike and stance.

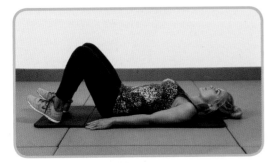

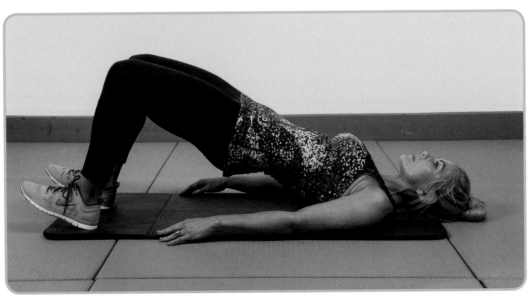

EXERCISE 82: HIP THRUST

- Set up in the position illustrated, with the bench lined up at the bottom of your shoulder blades (your back hinges on the bench at the line just beneath your shoulder blades – do not slide up and down the bench during the exercise).
- Place your feet so that your shins are vertical at the top of the hip thrust (your toes can be pointing straight ahead or turned out slightly – at 5 to 1 or 10 to 2, whichever is most comfortable).
- Drive through your heels and focus on using the glutes to push the hips straight up. Finish the movement with your hips as high as possible while maintaining a neutral spine.
- Use a steady controlled tempo throughout the exercise.

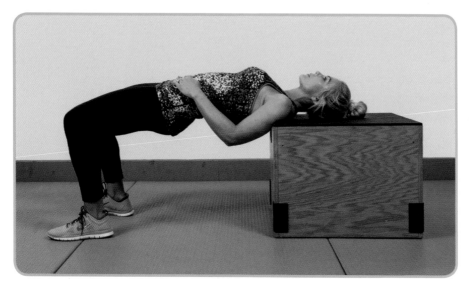

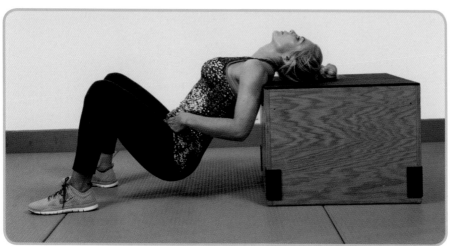

VERTICAL PUSH

EXERCISE 83: BARBELL SHOULDER PRESS

- Stand with your feet shoulder-width apart, holding the bar at your shoulders with a shoulder-width grip.
- Press the bar overhead (tuck in your chin as the bar passes your face to keep it out of the way!)
- When the bar passes your head, press it up and slightly backwards so that it ends up in line with the crown of your head.
- Lower the bar under control back down to your shoulders.

> Avoid arching your back and looking up at the bar.

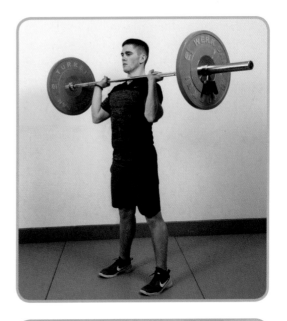

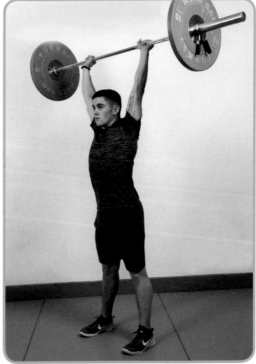

EXERCISE 84: DUMBBELL SHOULDER PRESS

- Stand with your feet hip-width apart and press both dumbbells overhead.
- Lower both dumbbells down to the shoulder (maintaining wrist over elbow).
- Return to the starting position by pressing the dumbbells back overhead.

This is a highly effective method for developing strength and stability through the shoulder complex. When you start to fatigue, you will naturally want to bend the arms when they are extended. Work hard – imagine you are holding the ceiling up with fully extended arms!

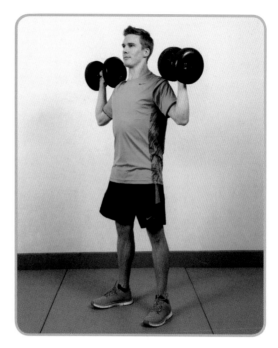

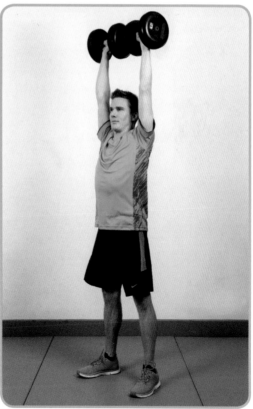

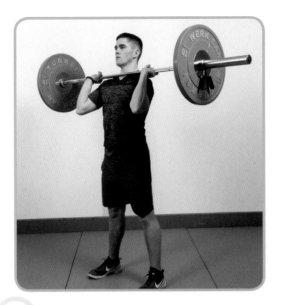

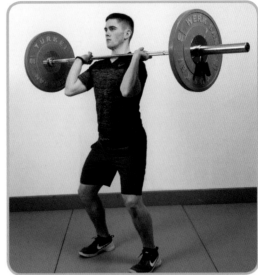

EXERCISE 85: PUSH PRESS

- Stand with your feet shoulder-width apart, holding the bar at your shoulders with a shoulder-width grip.
- Dip down until you are in a quarter-squat position, then immediately drive with your legs and allow the momentum generated to help you press the bar overhead (tuck in your chin as the bar passes your face to keep it out of the way!)
- When the bar passes your head, press it up and slightly backwards so that it ends up in line with the crown of your head.
- You will finish with the bar overhead and your arms and legs straight.
- Lower the bar under control back down to your shoulders.

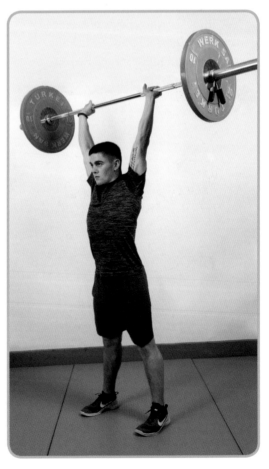

This exercise is pretty much the same as a barbell and dumbbell shoulder press but the lower body involvement allows you to lift heavier loads.

HORIZONTAL PUSH

EXERCISE 86: PUSH-UP

- Start with your hands slightly wider than shoulder-width apart. Tighten up through your core, ensuring that your back is flat.

- Lower your body until your chest is about 1cm (1½ inch) from the floor.
- Drive up to the starting position, where your arms will be completely extended.

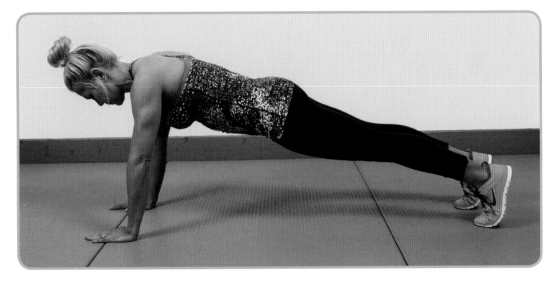

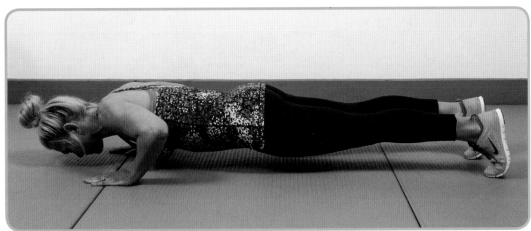

Variations

The push-up, when performed properly, is a really shoulder-friendly exercise but you need to make sure that your elbows are tucked to a 45-degree angle to the body. You may find this position tough to begin with, but your shoulders will thank you in the long run. There is an almost infinite number of variations; here are three of my favourites.

- **Incline** – changing the angle increases the load, making this a great progression.
- **Decline** – makes the exercise easier and is a great starting point.
- **Offset** – this is an excellent variation when you want to develop some more specific pushing strength.

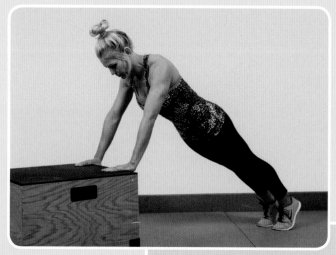

Push-up: incline

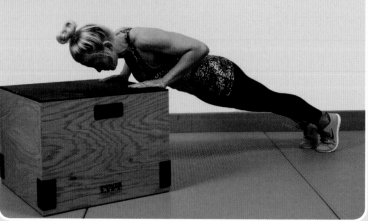

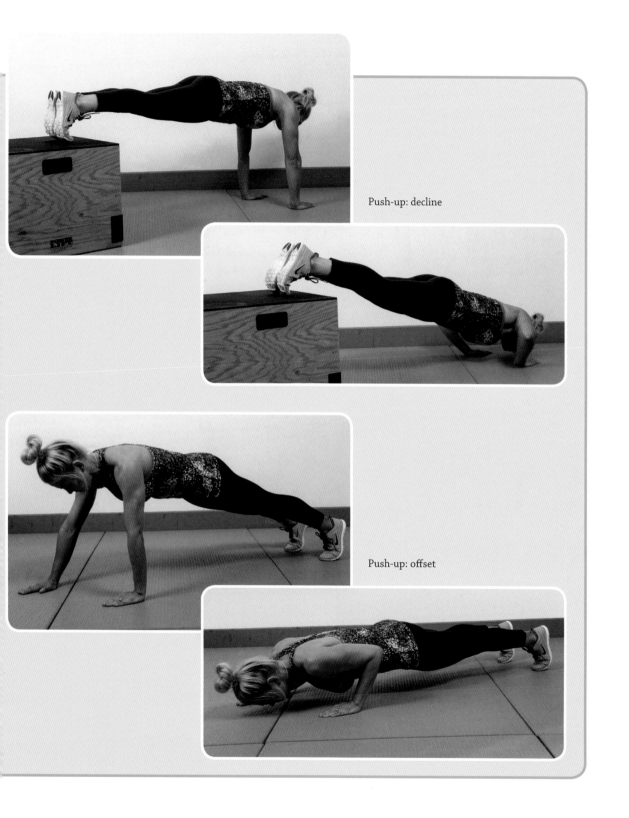

Push-up: decline

Push-up: offset

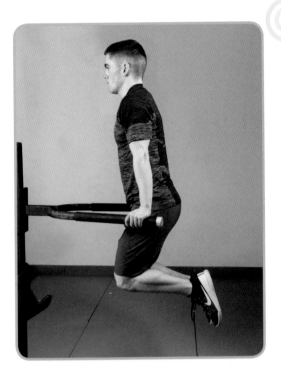

EXERCISE 87: DIP

- Support your bodyweight in an upright position, arms straight, hands gripping the dipping station.
- Lower your body by bending at the elbows.
- Keep your shoulders tucked close to your sides.
- Drive upwards until your arms are fully extended and you have returned to the starting position.

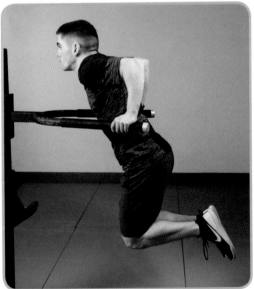

Variations

You can use heavy-duty superbands (create a loop by attaching the band to the chin-up bar and then sliding your knees into the loop – the elastic will stretch and offer assistance as you drive up towards the starting position) or, if you have access to a chin-up machine at your gym, that can be a useful alternative. To make dips harder, simply add an external load.

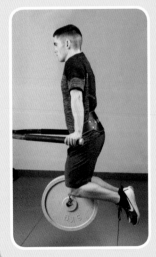

Dip: external load

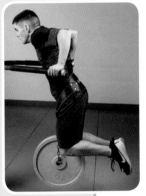

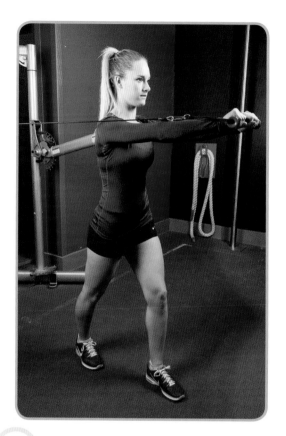 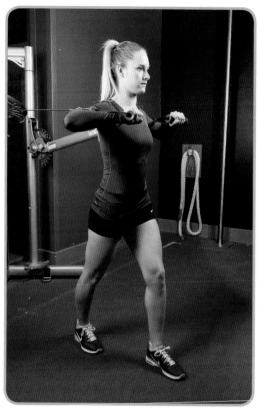

EXERCISE 88: CABLE CHEST PRESS

- Adopt a split stance with the front knee slightly bent (triple flexion: hip, ankle and knee) with your feet facing away from the cable machine and holding the cable handles in line with your chest.
- Extend both arms in front of your body.

Upper-body strength is an important component of physical fitness and is vital in transfering forces around the body. You can perform this exercise using one arm at a time – this increases the demand on your upper body as well as challenging your core.

EXERCISE 89: ALTERNATE DUMBBELL BENCH PRESS

- Lie on a flat bench, making sure you have five points of contact (left foot, right foot, hips, shoulders, head).
- Extend both arms above your chest.
- Lower one dumbbell to the side of the upper chest and then drive it back up.
- Repeat on the opposite side.

This is a highly effective method for developing strength and stability through the upper body. When you start to fatigue, you will naturally want to bend the elbow of the arm that is extended. Imagine you are holding the ceiling up with the extended arm!

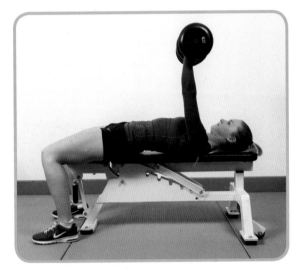

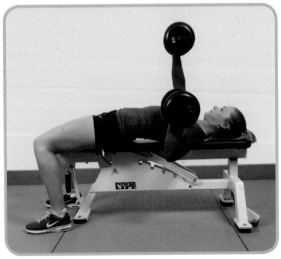

VERTICAL PULL

EXERCISE 90: CHIN-UP

- Take hold of the bar using a supinated grip (palms facing your body), with your hands just narrower than shoulder-width.
- Make sure you are in a complete straight 'hang' position.
- Drive your elbows down and back, to raise your body until your chin is above the bar.
- Reverse the movement under control to return to the starting position.

> You can make this exercise easier by using an assisted chin-up machine or heavy-duty superbands. Don't be tempted to perform partial repetitions, as it is important that you develop strength through a full ROM.

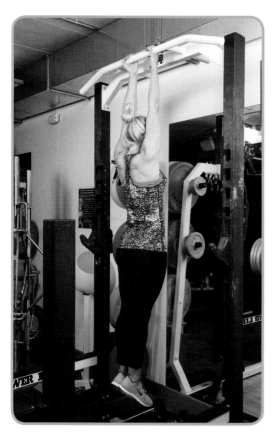

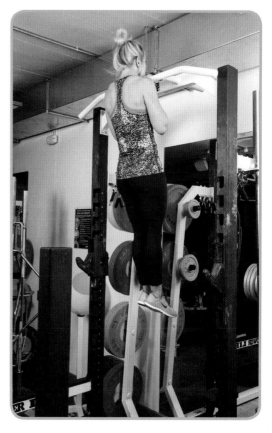

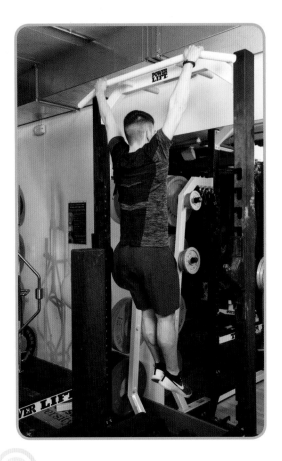
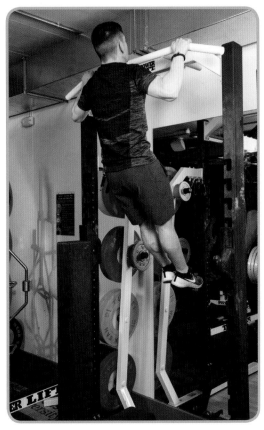

EXERCISE 91: PULL-UP

- Take hold of the bar using a pronated grip (palms facing away from your body), with your hands just outside shoulder-width.
- Make sure you are in a complete straight 'hang' position.
- Drive your elbows out and down to raise your body until your chin is above the bar.
- Reverse the movement under control to return to the starting position.

You can make this exercise easier by using an assisted chin-up machine or heavy-duty superbands. Don't be tempted to perform partial repetitions, as it is important that you develop strength through a full ROM.

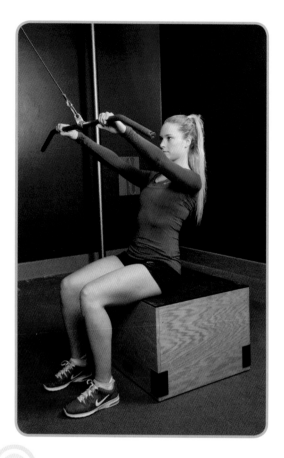
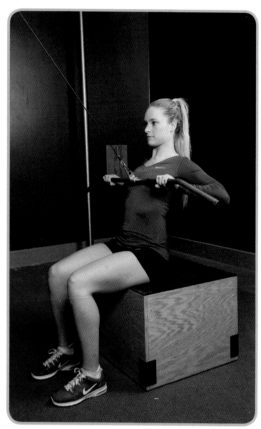

EXERCISE 92: LAT PULL-DOWN

- Sit in the lat pull-down machine so that your knees are at right angles and your feet are flat on the floor.
- Grip the bar using a wide grip (you can use a range of grips to bring about different training adaptations) and maintain correct upper body posture with your shoulders back and your chest up and out.
- Pull the bar to the top of your chest.
- Return the bar to the starting position by extending your arms.

This exercise has fallen out of fashion recently but it's still an excellent vertical pulling exercise that can be particularly useful when you don't have access to a chin-up bar or you need to establish some vertical pulling volume before attempting pull-ups and chin-ups.

HORIZONTAL PULL

EXERCISE 93: INVERSE PULL

- Hang underneath the bar with a pronated grip, your arms and legs fully extended and your body rigid.
- Set your shoulder blades.
- Pull up so your chest almost touches the bar (mid chest line).
- Lower back down to the starting position.

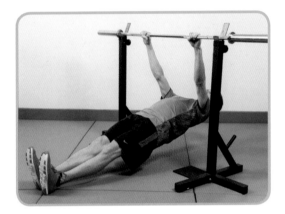

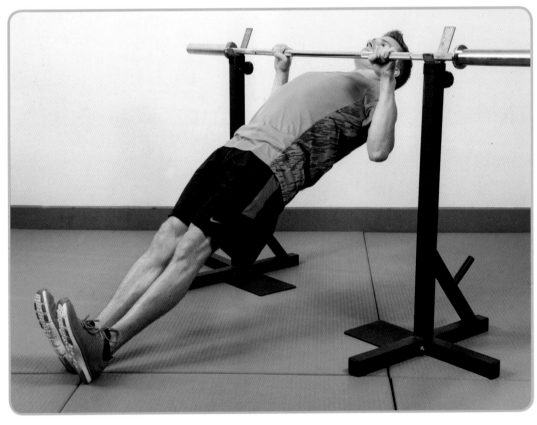

This exercise has four levels of difficulty

··

- Level One – Feet flat on the floor, knees bent (knees, hips and shoulders in alignment, forming a 'table top')
- Level Two – Legs fully extended
- Level Three – Feet raised on to a box or bench
- Level Four – Feet raised onto a stability ball.

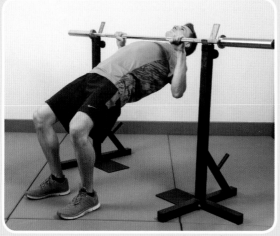

Level One

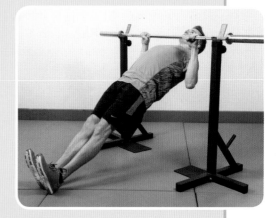

Level Two

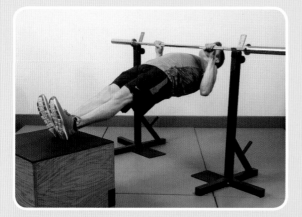

Level Three

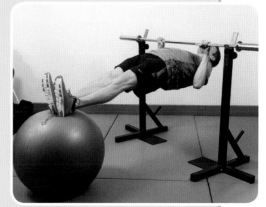

Level Four

EXERCISE 94: BAND/CABLE STANDING ROW

- Stand in an athletic position (triple flexion: hip, knee, ankle), with your feet about hip-width apart.
- Pull the band/cable towards you until the handle makes contact with your lower ribcage.
- Under control, return to the starting position.

> This exercise can be performed using a variety of resistance training equipment, ranging from resistance bands through to cable stacks.

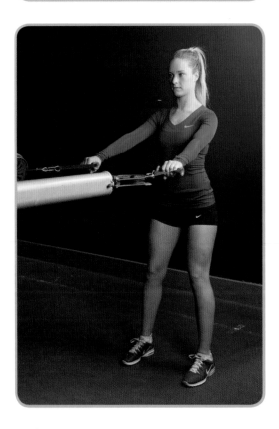
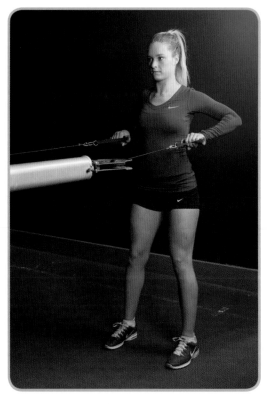

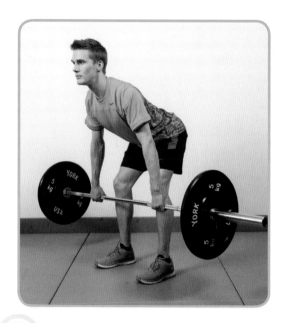
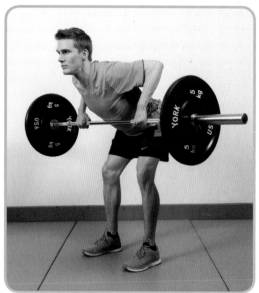

EXERCISE 95: BARBELL BENT-OVER ROW

- Stand with your feet hip-width apart, your knees slightly bent and your torso bent forwards at the hips to at least a 45-degree angle (maintaining a flat lower back).
- Hold the barbell in a pronated grip (your thumbs should just be brushing the outside of your thighs).
- Row the bar up to the ribcage and then lower back to the starting position, maintaining good posture throughout the lift.

Poor posture is a common issue and muscles in the upper back can often become deconditioned, leading to bad posture, poor mechanics and increased injury potential. Horizontal pulling exercises are an excellent way to improve the function of the upper back muscles and help reduce common shoulder injuries.

EXERCISE 96: DUMBBELL BENT-OVER ROW

- Stand with your feet hip-width apart, your knees slightly bent and your torso bent forwards at the hips to at least a 45-degree angle. Hold the dumbbells in a pronated grip (thumbs in, elbows out).
- Row both dumbbells up to the ribcage and then lower back to the starting position.

> This exercise can also be performed by alternating the dumbbells in a similar manner to the alternate dumbbell bench press (see p. 226).

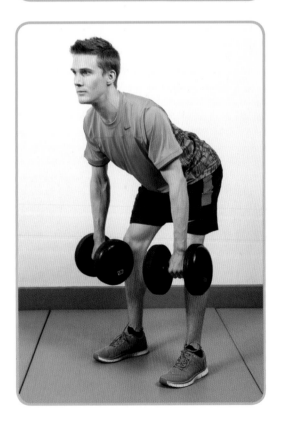
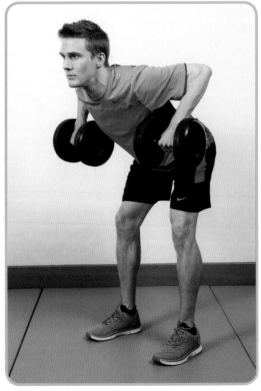

EXERCISE 97: 2-POINT DUMBBELL BENT-OVER ROW

- Start with your feet hip-width apart, then move into an offset stance with your left foot slightly staggered behind the right foot.
- Take up the same position as you would for a bent-over row, holding a dumbbell in your left hand.
- Row the dumbell up to your ribcage and then return to the starting position
- Repeat all repetitions in a set and then switch sides.

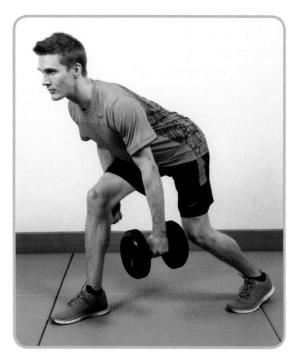

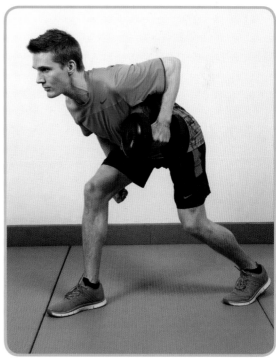

EXERCISE 98: SINGLE-ARM BARBELL ROW

- Place one end of an Olympic bar into the corner of a wall.
- Stand with the bar on your right-hand side, in a split stance (left leg forwards) and hold the bar with your right hand close to

- the collar (where the weight plates would normally sit.
- Take up the same position as you would for a bent-over row and perform the row.
- Repeat all repetitions before changing sides,

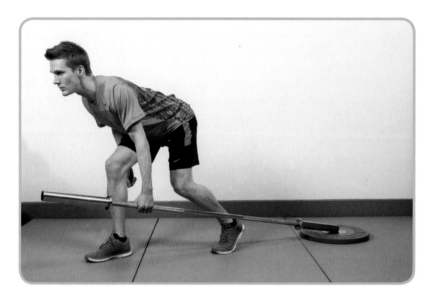

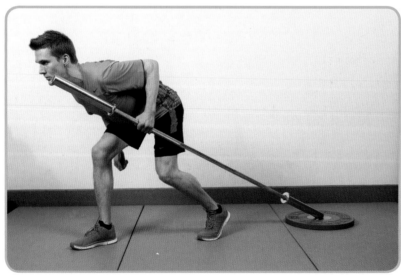

Variation

You can increase the load by placing weight plates on the end of the Olympic bar.

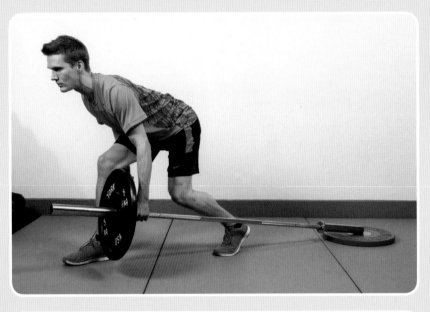

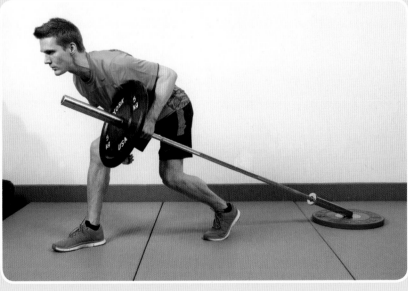

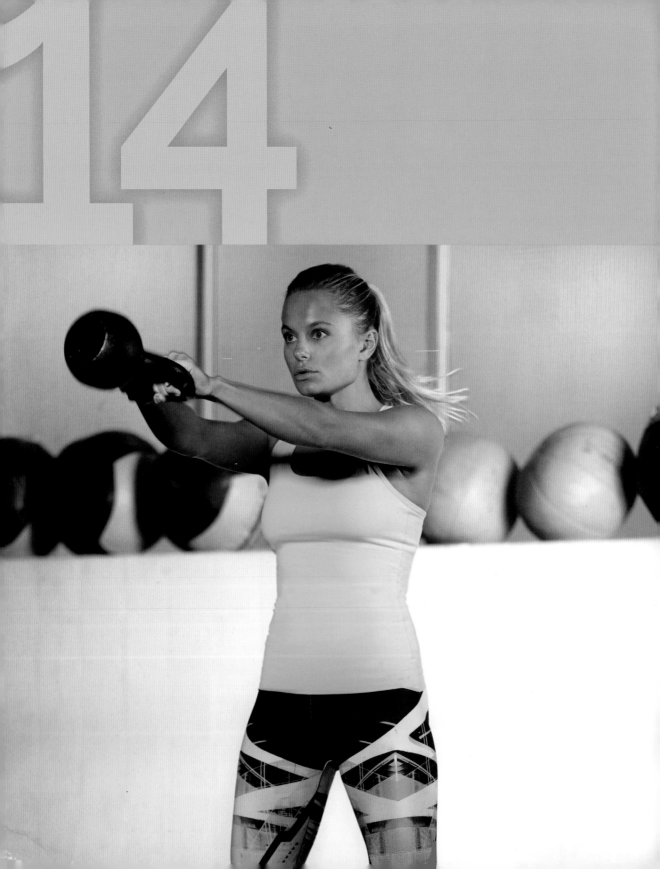

METABOLIC CONDITIONING

EXERCISE 99: MOUNTAIN CLIMBERS

- Start in a push-up position and drive one knee into your chest so you are balancing on both hands and one foot.
- Immediately switch the position of the legs by driving the first leg back to the starting position while bringing the opposite leg up to your chest.

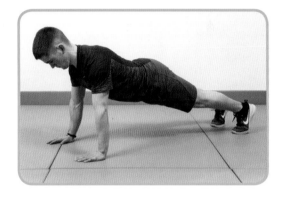

One repetition is a complete cycle of right and left legs. You should always have one foot off the floor. Make it easier – use a box for support.

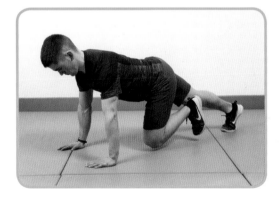

EXERCISE 100: SQUAT AND PRESS

- Take up the same starting position used for squats.
- Hold a weight (dumbbells, medicine ball, kettlebell, plate) at your shoulders.
- Drop into a squat and then drive back up.
- Press the weight overhead as you drive up from the bottom of the squat.

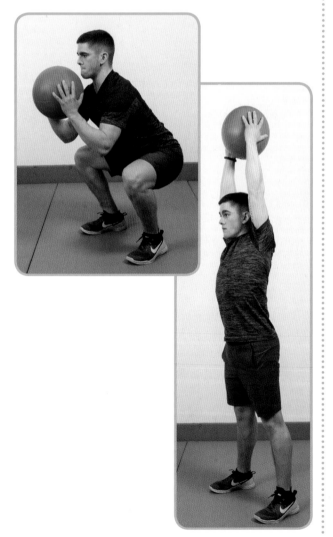

EXERCISE 101: SQUAT JUMPS

- Squat down into a half-squat position and immediately explode upwards, jumping as high as possible.
- Land under control by bending the knees and then dropping back into the half-squat position without pausing.

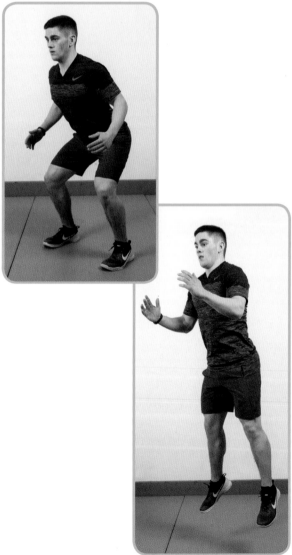

EXERCISE 102: BURPEES

- Start with your hands at your hips, squat down and place your hands on the floor.
- Drive your legs out behind your body until you are in the same position as the start of a push-up.
- Immediately jump your legs back underneath the body.
- Immediately jump back up to the starting position.

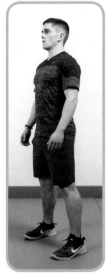
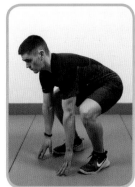
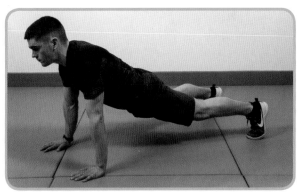
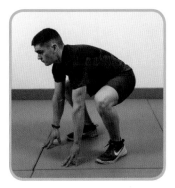
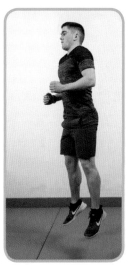

EXERCISE 103: KB SWINGS

- Hold a kettlebell with both hands. Adopt an athletic position.
- Bend forwards from the hips so that your forearms are in contact with your inner thighs.
- Swing the weight upwards and out in front of you, using the extension of your hips to move the load.
- Return to the starting position and repeat.

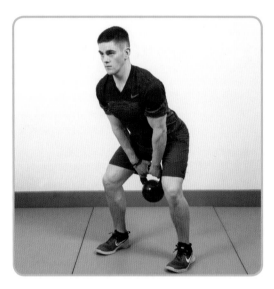

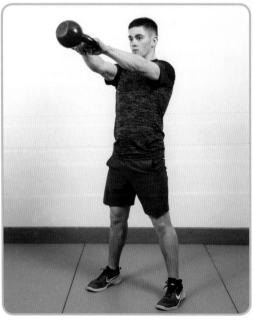

Variation

Hold the kettle-bell in one hand and when you reach the top of the movement, switch hands and return to the starting position – 1 repetition is a swing with both arms.

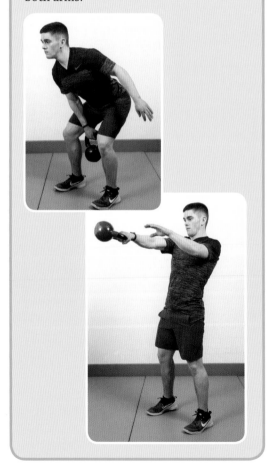

EXERCISE 104: SPLIT JUMPS (AKA SPLIT SQUAT SCREAMERS!)

- Start in a split squat position with one leg forwards and one leg back.
- Drop into a deep split squat and immediately explode off the floor.
- Land in the same position and immediately jump again.

> You can make this exercise more challenging by switching feet while in the air so that each landing is with a different foot at the front.

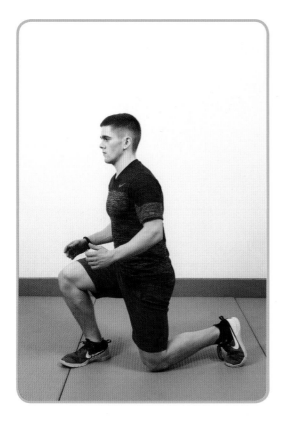

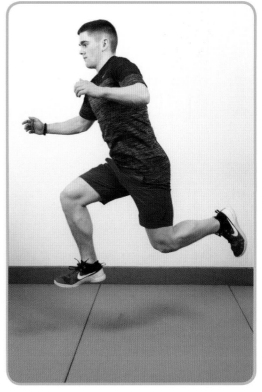

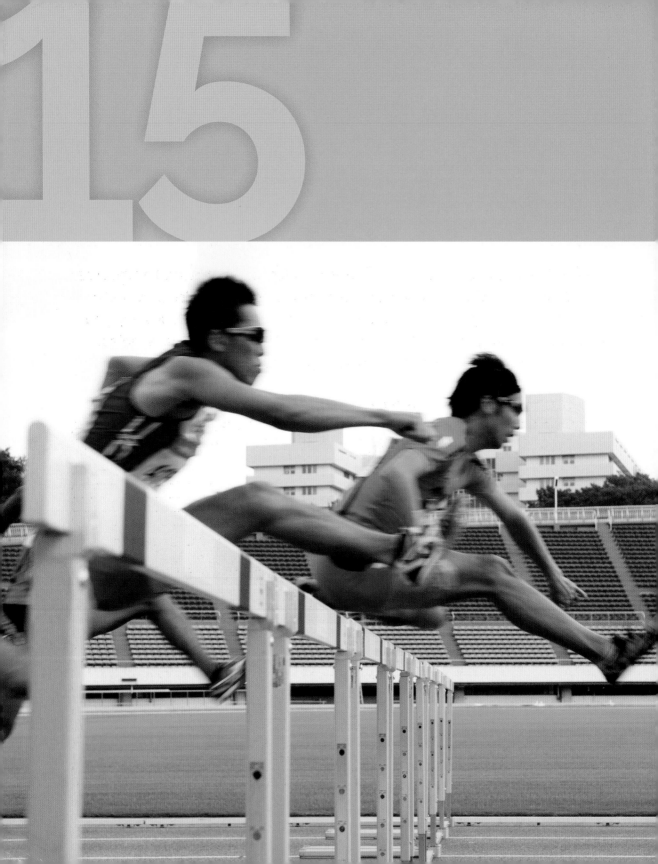

PROGRAMME TEMPLATES AND EXERCISE MATRIX

■ In this chapter I've provided you with programme templates for single, weekly and four-weekly sessions (pp.245-7). I've also provided a 16-week, 4 stage plan as well as an exercise matrix so you can develop your own training programmes. You can find printable versions of these tables online at www.bloomsbury.com/9781472908971.

Physical Preparation Programme – 1-session

INJURY REDUCTION			
Order	Exercise	Sets/Reps	Coaching Cue
1			
2			
3			
4			
5			
6			

MOVEMENT QUALITY			
Order	Exercise	Sets/Reps	Coaching Cue
1			
2			
3			
4			
5			
6			

STRENGTH AND POWER					
Order	Exercise	Coaching Cue	Sets/Reps	Tempo	Recovery
1					
2					
3					
4					
5					
6					

STRENGTH AND POWER - RECORD SHEET			Date:			
Order	Exercise	Sets/Reps	Load			
1						
2						
3						
4						
5						
6						

Physical Preparation Programme – 1-week

INJURY REDUCTION

Order	Exercise	Sets/Reps	Coaching Cue
1			
2			
3			
4			
5			
6			

MOVEMENT QUALITY

Order	Exercise	Sets/Reps	Coaching Cue
1			
2			
3			
4			
5			
6			

STRENGTH AND POWER – 1

Order	Exercise	Coaching Cue	Sets/Reps	Tempo	Recovery
1					
2					
3					
4					
5					
6					

STRENGTH AND POWER – 2

Order	Exercise	Coaching Cue	Sets/Reps	Tempo	Recovery
1					
2					
3					
4					
5					
6					

STRENGTH AND POWER 1: RECORD SHEET

Date:

Order	Exercise	Sets/Reps	Load
1			
2			
3			
4			
5			
6			

STRENGTH AND POWER 2: RECORD SHEET

Date:

Order	Exercise	Sets/Reps	Load
1			
2			
3			
4			
5			
6			

Physical Preparation Programme – 4-weeks

INJURY REDUCTION

Order	Exercise	Sets/Reps	Coaching Cue
1			
2			
3			
4			
5			
6			

MOVEMENT QUALITY

Order	Exercise	Sets/Reps	Coaching Cue
1			
2			
3			
4			
5			
6			

STRENGTH AND POWER – 1

Order	Exercise	Coaching Cue	Sets/Reps	Tempo	Recovery
1					
2					
3					
4					
5					
6					

STRENGTH AND POWER – 2

Order	Exercise	Coaching Cue	Sets/Reps	Tempo	Recovery
1					
2					
3					
4					
5					
6					

STRENGTH AND POWER 1: RECORD SHEET

Order	Exercise	Sets/Reps	Date:		Date:		Date:		Date:		Date:	
			Load	Load	Load	Load	Load	Load	Load	Load	Load	Load
1												
2												
3												
4												
5												
6												

STRENGTH AND POWER 2: RECORD SHEET

Order	Exercise	Sets/Reps	Date:		Date:		Date:		Date:		Date:	
			Load	Load	Load	Load	Load	Load	Load	Load	Load	Load
1												
2												
3												
4												
5												
6												

Physical Preparation Programme (Weeks 1–4)

INJURY REDUCTION

Order	Exercise	Sets/Reps	Coaching Cue
1	Myofascial Release	-	focus on key areas
2	Flexibility and Mobility	-	focus on key areas
3	Flutters	8-8-8	controlled movement
4	Mini-band Lateral Step	10-10 ea	athletic position, lead with knee
5	Calf Raise	10-10-10	controlled movement
6			

MOVEMENT QUALITY TRAINING

Order	Exercise	Sets/Reps	Coaching Cue
1	Plank	30-60s	brace
2	Side Hold	15-45s ea	brace
3	Aleknas	5-5-5	controlled movement
4	Single-leg	30-60s ea	stay compact
5	X-Band Walks	10-10 ea	maintain posture
6			

STRENGTH AND POWER – 1

Order	Exercise	Coaching Cue	Sets/Reps	Tempo	Recovery
1	Front Squat	controlled movement	8-8-8-8	2 1 1	60s
2	Romanian Deadlift	flat back	8-8-8-8	2 1 1	60s
3	Hip Thrust	squeeze gluteals at the top	10-10-10	1 1 1	60s
4	Push-up	maintain postural alignment	10-10-8-8	2 1 2	60s
5	Inverse Pull	full range of motion	5-5-5-5	1 1 1	60s
6	Chin-up	full range of motion	5-5-5-5	1 0 1	60s

STRENGTH AND POWER – 2

Order	Exercise	Coaching Cue	Sets/Reps	Tempo	Recovery
1	Split Squat	maintain upright torso	8-8-8 ea	1 1 1	60s
2	Lying Hip Extension	squeeze gluteal at the top	10-10-10	1 1 1	60s
3	Push-up	maintain postural alignment	10-10-8-8	2 1 2	60s
4	Inverse Pull	full range of motion	5-5-5-5	1 1 1	60s
5	Chin-up	full range of motion	5-5-5-5	1 0 1	60s
6	DB Shoulder Press	full range of motion	8-8-5-5	1 0 1	60s

STRENGTH AND POWER 1: RECORD SHEET

Order	Exercise	Sets/Reps	Date:	Date:	Date:	Date:
			Load	Load	Load	Load
1	Front Squat	8-8-8-8				
2	Romanian Deadlift	8-8-8-8				
3	Hip Thrust	10-10-10				
4	Push-up	10-10-8-8				
5	Inverse Pull	5-5-5-5				
6	Chin-up	5-5-5-5				

STRENGTH AND POWER 2: RECORD SHEET

Order	Exercise	Sets/Reps	Date:	Date:	Date:	Date:
			Load	Load	Load	Load
1	Split Squat	8-8-8 ea				
2	Lying Hip Extension	10-10-10				
3	Push-up	10-10-8-8				
4	Inverse Pull	5-5-5-5				
5	Chin-up	5-5-5-5				
6	DB Shoulder Press	8-8-5-5				

Physical Preparation Programme (Weeks 5–8)

INJURY REDUCTION

Order	Exercise	Sets/Reps	Coaching Cue
1	Myofascial Release	-	focus on key areas
2	Flexibility and Mobility	-	focus on key areas
3	YTWL	8 ea	controlled movement
4	Lying Hip Abduction	5-5-5	controlled movement
5	Calf Raise	10-10-10	controlled movement
6			

MOVEMENT QUALITY TRAINING

Order	Exercise	Sets/Reps	Coaching Cue
1	Plank	60-90s	brace
2	Side Hold	60-90 ea	brace
3	Aleknas	10-10	controlled movement
4	Single-leg Balance abd Reach	5-5 ea	stay compact
5	X-Band Walks	10-10-10 ea	maintain posture
6			

STRENGTH AND POWER – 1

Order	Exercise	Coaching Cue	Sets/Reps	Tempo	Recovery
1	Front Squat	controlled movement	8-8-5-5	2 1 1	60s
2	Romanian Deadlift	flat back	8-8-8-8	2 1 1	60s
3	Hip Thrust	squeeze gluteals at the top	10-10-10	1 1 1	60s
4	DB Alt Bench Press	controlled movement	8-8-8-8 ea	2 1 2	60s
5	DB Bent-over Row	flat back	8-8-8-8 ea	1 1 1	60s
6	Chin-up	full range of motion	5-5-5-5	1 0 1	60s

STRENGTH AND POWER – 2

Order	Exercise	Coaching Cue	Sets/Reps	Tempo	Recovery
1	Bulgarian Split Squat	maintain upright torso	8-8-8 ea	1 1 1	60s
2	Split RDL	squeeze gluteasl at the top	10-10-10	1 1 1	60s
3	Inverse Pull	full range of motion	5-5-5-5	1 1 1	60s
4	Chin-up	full range of motion	5-5-5-5	1 0 1	60s
5	DB Shoulder Press	full range of motion	8-8-5-5	1 0 1	60s
6					

STRENGTH AND POWER 1: RECORD SHEET

Order	Exercise	Sets/Reps	Date: Load	Date: Load	Date: Load	Date: Load
1	Front Squat	8-8-5-5				
2	Romanian Deadlift	8-8-8-8				
3	Hip Thrust	10-10-10				
4	DB Alt Bench Press	8-8-8-8 ea				
5	DB Bent-over Row	8-8-8-8 ea				
6	Chin-up	5-5-5-5				

STRENGTH AND POWER 2: RECORD SHEET

Order	Exercise	Sets/Reps	Date: Load	Date: Load	Date: Load	Date: Load
1	Bulgarian Split Squat	8-8-8 ea				
2	Split RDL	10-10-10				
3	Inverse Pull	5-5-5-5				
4	Chin-up	5-5-5-5				
5	DB Shoulder Press	5-5-5-5				
6						

Physical Preparation Programme (Weeks 9–12)

INJURY REDUCTION

Order	Exercise	Sets/Reps	Coaching Cue
1	Myofascial Release	-	focus on key areas
2	Flexibility and Mobility	-	focus on key areas
3	Shoulder Shuffles	30s–30s	controlled movement
4	Mini-band Hip Activation	5 ea	maintain posture
5	Ankle Jumps	10-10-10	explosive
6			

MOVEMENT QUALITY TRAINING

Order	Exercise	Sets/Reps	Coaching Cue
1	Aleknas	60-90s	brace
2	Bird Dog	60-90 ea	brace
3	Barbell Roll Out	10-10	controlled movement
4	Single-leg Balance and Reach	5-5 ea	stay compact
5	Big X-Band Walks	10-10-10 ea	maintain posture
6			

STRENGTH AND POWER – 1

Order	Exercise	Coaching Cue	Sets/Reps	Tempo	Recovery
1	Push Press	dip and drive	5-5-5-5 ea	X	120s
2	Front Squat	controlled movement	5-5-5-5	1 0 X	120s
3	Romanian Deadlift	flat back	5-5-5-5	1 0 X	120s
4	DB Bench Press	maintain postural alignment	8-8-5-5 ea	2 1 2	90s
5	Single-arm Bent-over Row	flat back	8-8-5-5 ea	1 1 1	90s
6	Chin-up	full range of motion	5-5-5-5	1 0 1	90s

STRENGTH AND POWER – 2

Order	Exercise	Coaching Cue	Sets/Reps	Tempo	Recovery
1	Lunge	maintain upright torso	8-8-8-8 ea	1 0 X	120s
2	Split RDL	squeeze gluteasl at the top	8-8-8-8 ea	1 1 1	120s
3	Inverse Pull	full range of motion	5-5-5-5	1 1 1	90s
4	Chin-up	full range of motion	5-5-5-5	1 0 1	60s
5	DB Shoulder Press	full range of motion	8-8-5-5	1 0 1	60s
6					

STRENGTH AND POWER 1: RECORD SHEET

Order	Exercise	Sets/Reps	Date: Load	Date: Load	Date: Load
1	Push Press	5-5-5-5 ea			
2	Front Squat	5-5-5-5			
3	Romanian Deadlift	5-5-5-5			
4	DB Bench Press	8-8-5-5 ea			
5	Single-arm Bent-over Row	8-8-5-5 ea			
6	Chin-up	5-5-5-5			

STRENGTH AND POWER 2: RECORD SHEET

Order	Exercise	Sets/Reps	Date: Load	Date: Load	Date: Load
1	Lunge	8-8-8-8 ea			
2	Split RDL	8-8-8-8 ea			
3	Inverse Pull	5-5-5-5			
4	Chin-up	5-5-5-5			
5	DB Shoulder Press	8-8-5-5			
6					

Physical Preparation Programme (Weeks 13–16)

INJURY REDUCTION

Order	Exercise	Sets/Reps	Coaching Cue
1	Myofascial Release	-	focus on key areas
2	Flexibility and Mobility	-	focus on key areas
3	Truck Drivers	5-5-5	controlled movement
4	Mini-band Step and Squat	10-10 ea	maintain posture
5	Ankle Hops	10-10-10 ea	explosive
6			

MOVEMENT QUALITY TRAINING

Order	Exercise	Sets/Reps	Coaching Cue
1	Standing Plate Rotations	10-10 ea	dynamic movement
2	Barbell Rotations	10-10 ea	dynamic movement
3	Barbell Roll Out	10-10	controlled movement
4	Single-leg Balance and Reach	5-5-5 ea	stay compact
5	Big X-Band Walks	10-10-10 ea	maintain posture
6			

STRENGTH AND POWER – 1

Order	Exercise	Coaching Cue	Sets/Reps	Tempo	Recovery
1	Front Squat	controlled movement	5-5-5-5	1 0 X	120s
2	Romanian Deadlift	flat back	5-5-5-5	1 0 X	120s
3	DB Bench Press	maintain postural alignment	5-5-5-5 ea	1 0 X	90s
4	Single-arm Bent-over Row	flat back	5-5-5-5 ea	X 0 1	90s
5	Chin-up	full range of motion	5-5-5	1 0 1	90s
6					

STRENGTH AND POWER – 2

Order	Exercise	Coaching Cue	Sets/Reps	Tempo	Recovery
1	Push Press	dip and drive	3-3-3-3 ea	X	120s
2	Step-up	maintain upright torso	5-5-5-5 ea	X 0 1	120s
3	Split RDL	squeeze gluteal at the top	5-5-5-5 ea	1 0 X	120s
4	Inverse Pull	full range of motion	5-5-5-5	1 1 1	90s
5	Chin-up	full range of motion	5-5-5	1 0 1	60s
6					

STRENGTH AND POWER 1: RECORD SHEET

Order	Exercise	Sets/Reps	Date: Load	Date: Load	Date: Load	Date: Load
1	Front Squat	5-5-5-5				
2	Romanian Deadlift	5-5-5-5				
3	DB Bench Press	5-5-5-5 ea				
4	Single-arm Bent-over Row	5-5-5-5 ea				
5	Chin-up	5-5-5				
6						

STRENGTH AND POWER 2: RECORD SHEET

Order	Exercise	Sets/Reps	Date: Load	Date: Load	Date: Load	Date: Load
1	Push Press	3-3-3 ea				
2	Step-up	5-5-5-5 ea				
3	Split RDL	5-5-5-5 ea				
4	Inverse Pull	5-5-5-5				
5	Chin-up	5-5-5				
6						

Exercise	Injury reduction			Movement Quality		Strength and Power						
	Lower leg, ankle, foot	Knee	Shoulder	Flexibility & Mobility	Body Control	Knee Dominant	Hip Dominant	Vertical Push	Horizontal Push	Vertical Pull	Horizontal Pull	Metabolic Conditioning
Calf Raise (Gastrocnemius)	X				X							
Calf Raise (Soleus)	X				X							
Eccentrics	X				X							
Ankle Jumps	X				X							
Single-leg Balance	X	X			X							
Ankle Drops	X			X	X							
Eccentric Knee Squat	X	X		X	X	X						
Dynamic Achilles Stretch	X	X			X							
Eccentric Reach	X			X	X							
Mini-band Lateral Step	X	X			X							
Mini-band Step and Squat	X	X			X							
Mini-band Hip Activation	X	X			X							
Lying Hip Abduction	X	X			X							
4-Point Hip Extension	X	X			X							
Bridge	X	X			X		X					
3-Point Bridge	X	X			X		X					
Single-leg Squats	X	X		X	X	X		X	X	X	X	
Shoulder Circle			X	X				X	X	X	X	
PNF Diagonal			X	X	X			X	X	X	X	
Figure 8			X	X	X			X	X	X	X	
RTWs			X	X	X			X	X	X	X	
Flutters			X		X			X	X	X	X	
Y T W L			X		X			X	X	X	X	
Truck Drivers			X		X			X	X	X	X	
Shoulder Shuffles			X		X			X	X	X	X	
X-Band Walks	X	X	X		X			X	X	X	X	
Big X-Band Walks	X	X	X		X			X	X	X	X	
Plantar Fascia Roll	X	X		X								
Calf Foam Roll	X	X		X								
Tibialis Anterior Foam Roll	X	X		X								
Gluteal Foam Roll	X	X		X								
Hamstring Foam Roll	X	X		X								
Quadriceps/Hip Flexors Foam Roll	X	X		X								
Iliotibial Band (ITB) Foam Roll	X	X		X								
Hip Flexors Foam Roll	X	X		X								
Lower Back/Quadratus Lumborum Foam Roll				X								
Thoracic Foam Roll			X	X								
Hamstring Stretch	X	X		X								
Hip Stretch	X	X		X								
Hip Flexors/Quadriceps Stretch	X	X		X								
Gluteal Stretch	X	X		X								
Gastrocnemius Stretch	X	X		X								
Soleus Stretch	X	X		X								
Back Stretch			X	X								
Chest Stretch			X	X								
Low Back Complex				X								
Hip Flexor Complex		X		X								
Gluteal Complex		X		X								
Hamstring Complex		X		X								
Giant Circle		X		X	X	X						
Romanian Deadlift		X		X	X		X					X
Squat		X		X	X	X						X

Exercise	Injury reduction			Movement Quality		Strength and Power						
	Lower leg, ankle, foot	Knee	Shoulder	Flexibility & Mobility	Body Control	Knee Dominant	Hip Dominant	Vertical Push	Horizontal Push	Vertical Pull	Horizontal Pull	Metabolic Conditioning
Lunge		X		X	X	X						X
Plank					X							
Side Holds					X							
Bird Dog					X							
Band/Cable Isometrics			X		X							
Barbell Roll Out			X		X							X
Aleknas			X		X							X
T Rotate and Hold			X	X	X							X
Get-ups					X							X
Band/Cable Rotations					X							X
Barbell Rotations					X							X
Seated Plate Rotations					X							X
Standing Plate Rotations					X							X
Medicine Ball Front Rotation Throw					X							X
Sngle-leg Balance	X	X			X							
Single-leg Balance and Reach	X	X			X							
Front Squat	X	X		X	X	X						X
Back Squat	X	X		X	X	X						X
Overhead Squat	X	X		X	X	X						X
Split Squat	X	X		X	X	X						X
Bulgarian Split Squat	X	X		X	X	X						X
Lunge	X	X		X	X	X						X
Step-up	X	X			X	X						X
Romanian Deadlift (RDL)	X	X		X	X		X					X
Split Romanian Deadlift (RDL)	X	X		X	X		X					X
Deadlift	X	X		X	X		X					X
Single-leg Deadlift	X	X		X	X		X					X
Lying Hip Extension	X	X			X		X					X
Hip Thrust	X	X			X		X					X
Barbell Shoulder Press			X		X			X				X
Dumbbell Shoulder Press			X		X			X				X
Push Press			X		X			X				X
Push-up			X		X				X			X
Dip			X		X				X			X
Cable Chest Press			X		X				X			X
Alternate Dumbbell Bench Press			X		X				X			X
Chin-up			X		X					X		X
Pull-up			X		X					X		X
Inverse Pull			X		X						X	X
Lat Pulldown			X		X					X		X
Band/Cable Standing Row			X		X						X	X
Barbell Bent Over Row			X		X						X	X
Dumbbell Bent-over Row			X		X						X	X
2-Point Dumbbell Bent-over Row			X		X						X	X
Single-arm Barbell Row			X		X						X	X
Mountain Climbers					X							X
Squat and Press	X	X	X	X	X	X						X
Squat Jumps	X	X			X	X						X
Burpees					X							X
KB Swings	X	X	X		X		X					X
Split Jumps	X	X			X	X						X

GLOSSARY

Adaptive response – the body's physiological response to a training stimulus

Aerobic system – metabolic system that requires oxygen to produces through the break down of food through a series of chemical reactions.

Anaerobic system – metabolic system that generates energy without the need for oxygen.

ATP-PC system – anaerobic energy system that generates energy from phosphocreatine stored in muscle cells

Bioenergetics – study of different cellular metabolic processes that can lead to production and utilisation of energy.

Biomechanics – application of physics and mechanics to the study of movement to develop an understanding of how the body produces force, and is affected by external forces.

Central adaptation – adaptations relating to the cardiovascular system.

Dorsiflex – movement of the foot and hand flexion so that the foot moves typically in an upwards direction.

Explosive strength – ability to move in one explosive movement or in a series of strong, sudden movements.

Force velocity curve – indicates the relationship between muscle tensions and the velocity of the shortening and lengthening of a muscle.

Functional capacity – High levels of fitness that provide the ability to function at a lower percentage of maximum capacity for any given stimulus.

Functional flexibility – appropriate levels of flexibility and mobility to allow smooth, unrestricted, pain free movement.

Fundamental movement skill – foundation movement patterns that involve different body parts that are the precursor patterns to the more specialised, complex skills used in sport and physical recreation.

Gross athleticism - result of athletic movement skills development that involves learning proper techniques for a wide range of fitness qualities, including strength and power, balance, coordination, flexibility and metabolic conditioning.

Homeostasis – regulation of internal functions within the body to keep conditions stable and relatively constant.

Hyperadaptation – adaptation to a training stimulus allowing the body to cope more efficiently with the training stimulus.

Hypertrophy – an increase in muscle tissue size due to an increase in the size of the functional cells.

Macrocycle – complete periodised plan that works towards peaking for a specific goal

Maximum strength – greatest force that can be exerted in a single maximum voluntary contraction (irrespective of body size or muscle size)

Mesocycle – phase of training (typically 2-6 weeks) where the training programme emphasises the same type of physical adaptations.

Metabolic conditioning – conditioning exercises intended to increase the storage and delivery of energy for any activity.

Microcycle - typically a 7-10 day training period.

Movement quality training – 4-step training process that can be used to prepare the body and develop fluid, athletic movement.

Multidimensional movement - movements in all planes of motion using multiple joints.

Neuromuscular control – interaction between the nervous and musculoskeletal systems to produce movement in response to a stimulus.

Periodisation – a structured programme that divides training into manageable phases.

Peripheral adaptation – adaptations relating to the neuromuscular system.

Phase potentiation - training a specific fitness quality to enhance gains in a different fitness quality during subsequent training phases.

Physiological adaptation - ongoing process by which body functions respond and adapt to stress of any kind.

Physiological stress – training stimulus (stressor) that is over and above habitual the level.

Progressive overload – progressive overloading of the body systems and fuel stores to provide sufficient stimulus to enhance physical, physiological and performance outcomes.

Reactive strength – ability to effectively use the stretch shortening cycle (SSC) – i.e. the ability to absorb impact (eccentric forces and explode rapidly from the impact with high levels of force (concentric contraction).

Reverse periodisation – training concept based on maintaining intensity closer to that of the demands of the activity whilst increasing training volume over time.

Self-myofascial release – soft tissue therapy that can release tension, eliminate pain and restore motion by applying sustained pressure into the myofascial connective tissue.

Speed of movement – speed at which each repetition is performed.

Strength endurance – ability to produce force over repeated efforts.

Superset – combination of two or more exercises (typically upper and lower body or different body parts) with all reps completed of both exercises together without resting.

Time under tension – length of time a muscle is under strain

Trigger point – localized palpable area of deep hypersensitivity, which, when irritated, results in pain being referred to another area, often coincides with a tight band or knot in the muscle or fascia.

INDEX